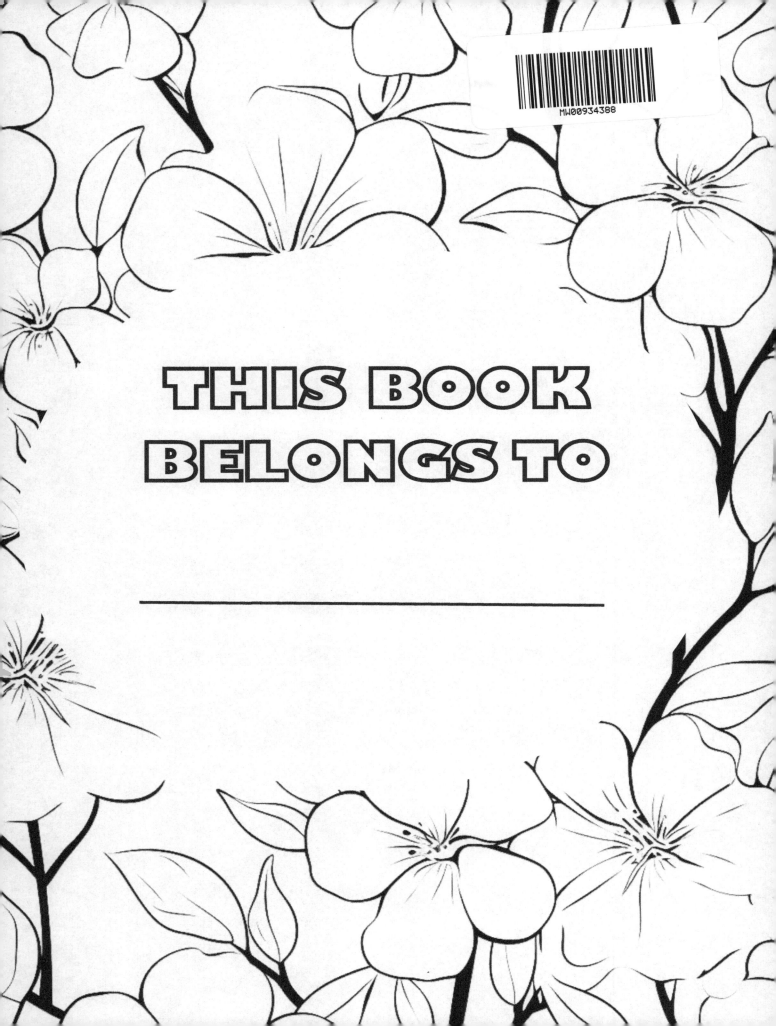

THIS BOOK
BELONGS TO

_____

Welcome to "Whispers of Motherhood"

Dear Beautiful Moms-in-Waiting,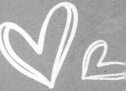

Step into a world where colors embrace inspiration!

We're thrilled to introduce "Whispers of Motherhood," a uniquely designed coloring book with quotes tailored to accompany you on this incredible journey

Celebrate impending motherhood as you blend hues and wisdom on every page.

Thank you for choosing "Whispers of Motherhood" for your creative moments.

Happy coloring, and may each stroke resonate with the joyful whispers of anticipation and love.

With warmth,
Stella Booker Publishing

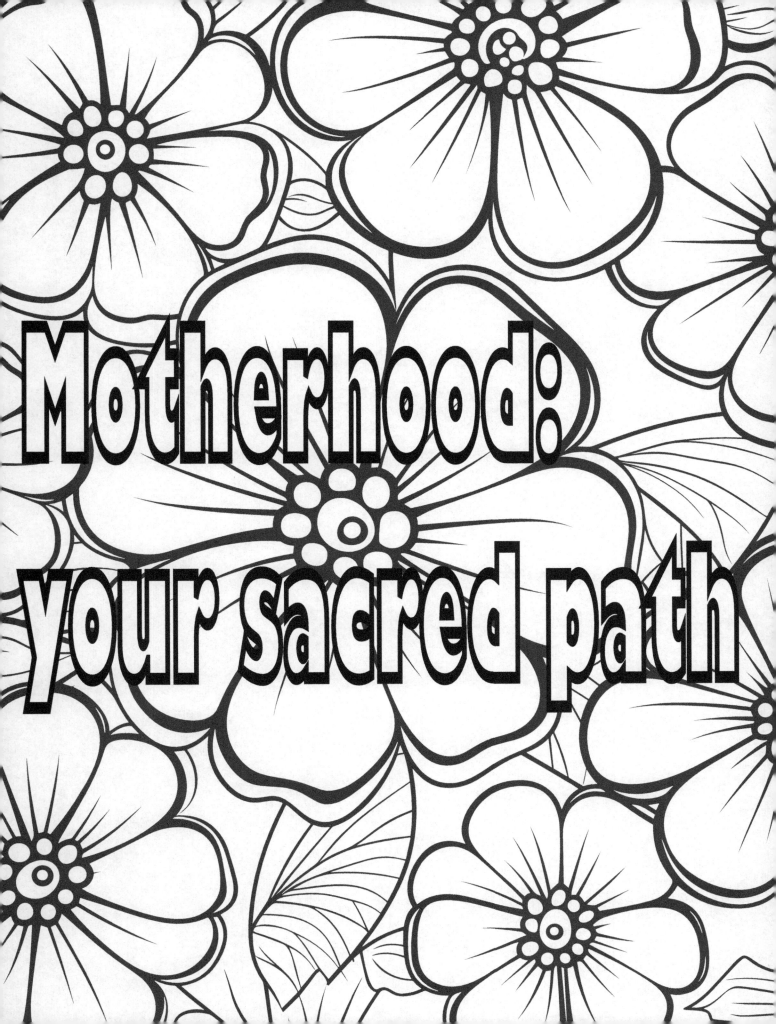

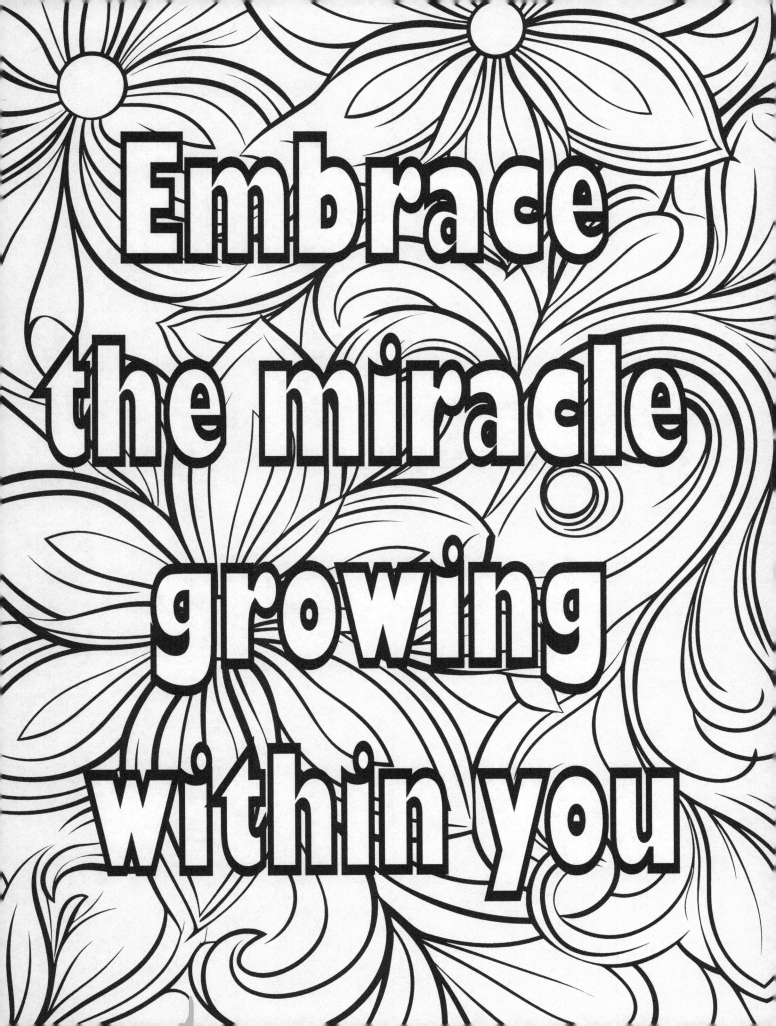

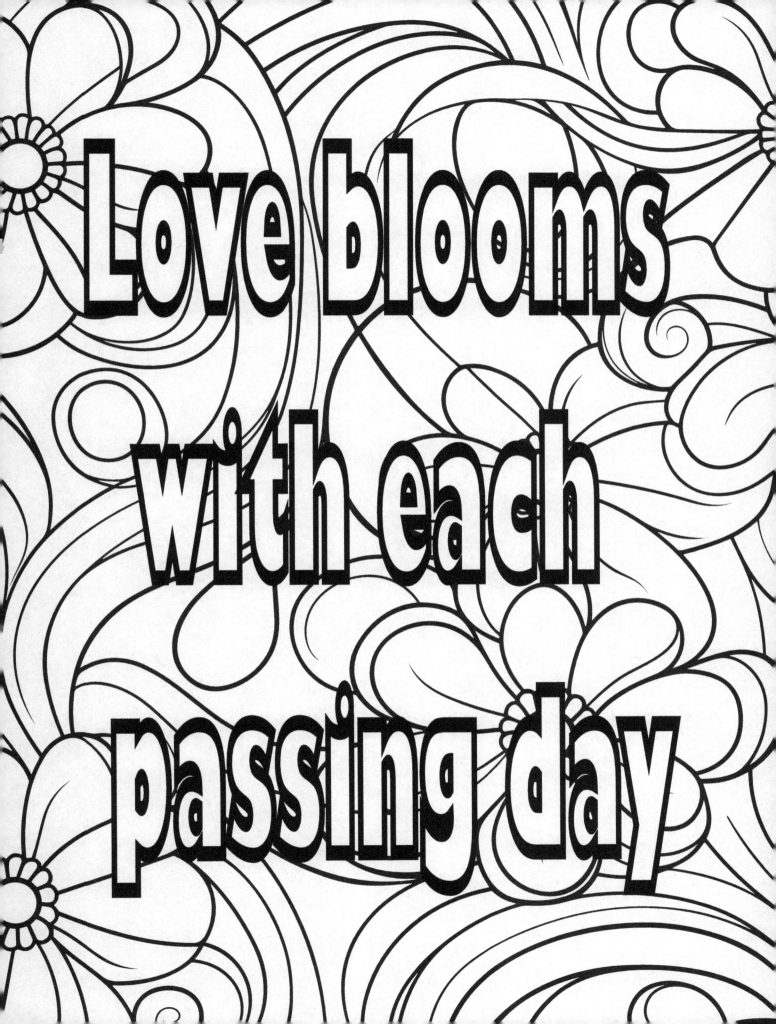

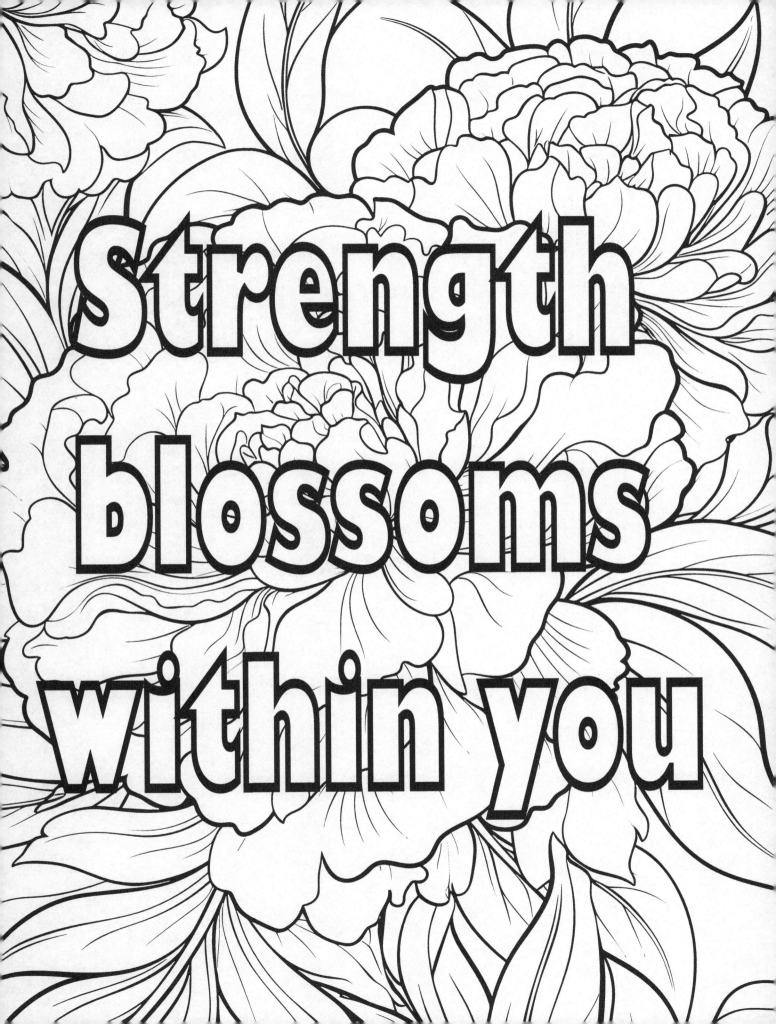

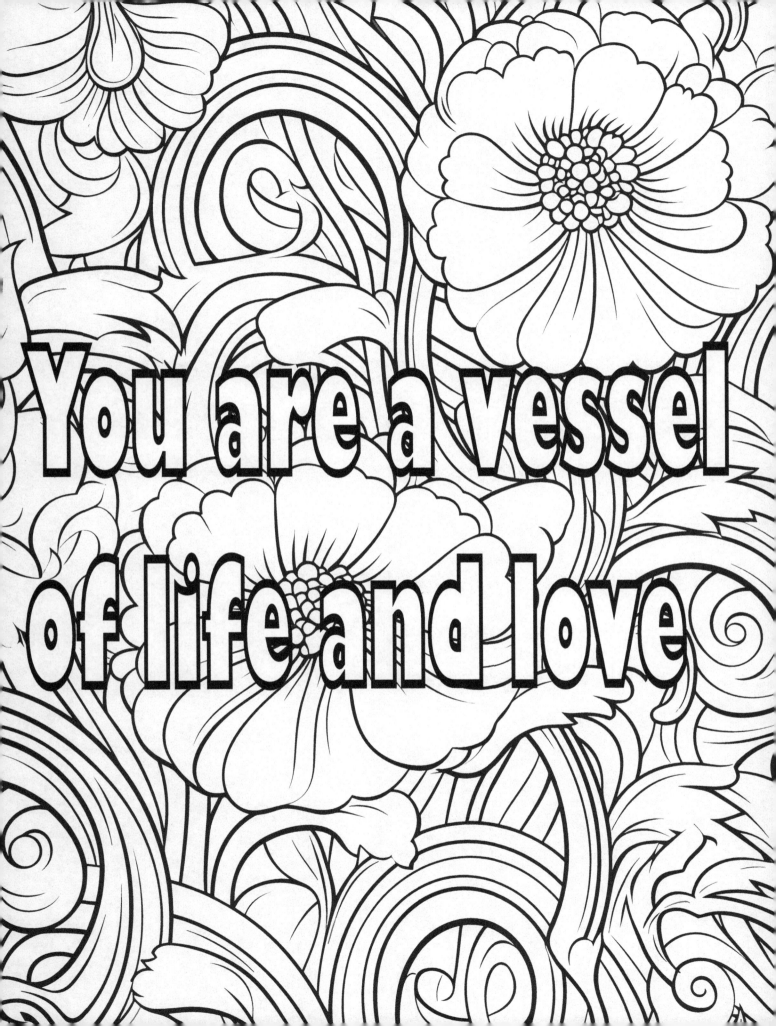

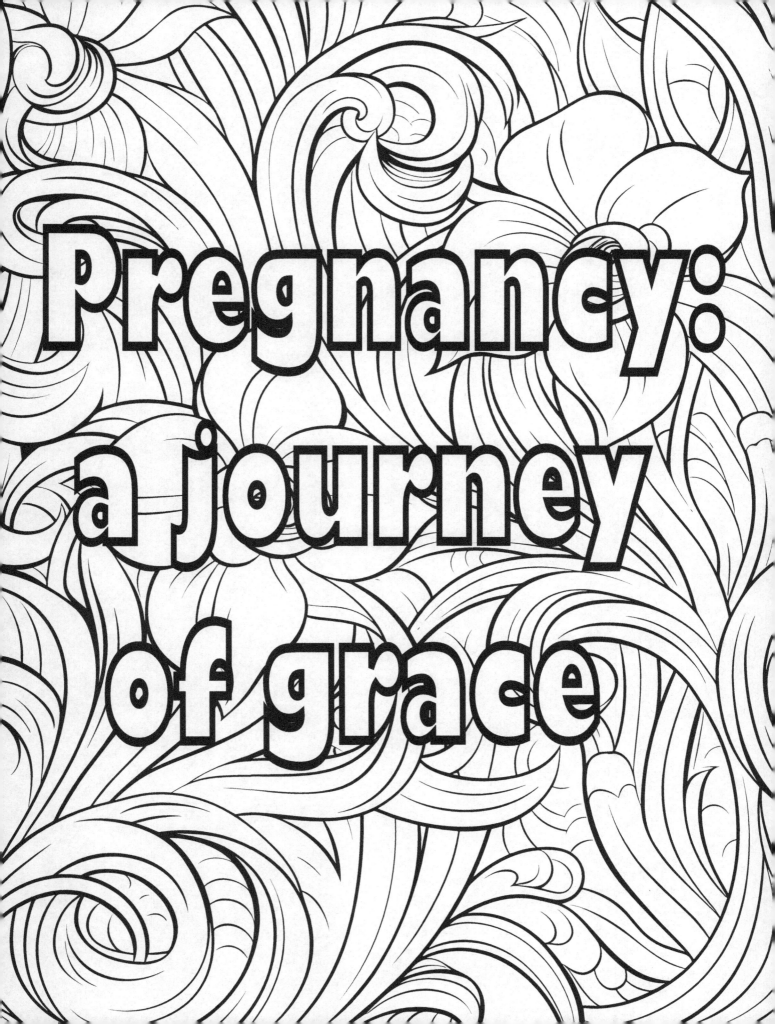

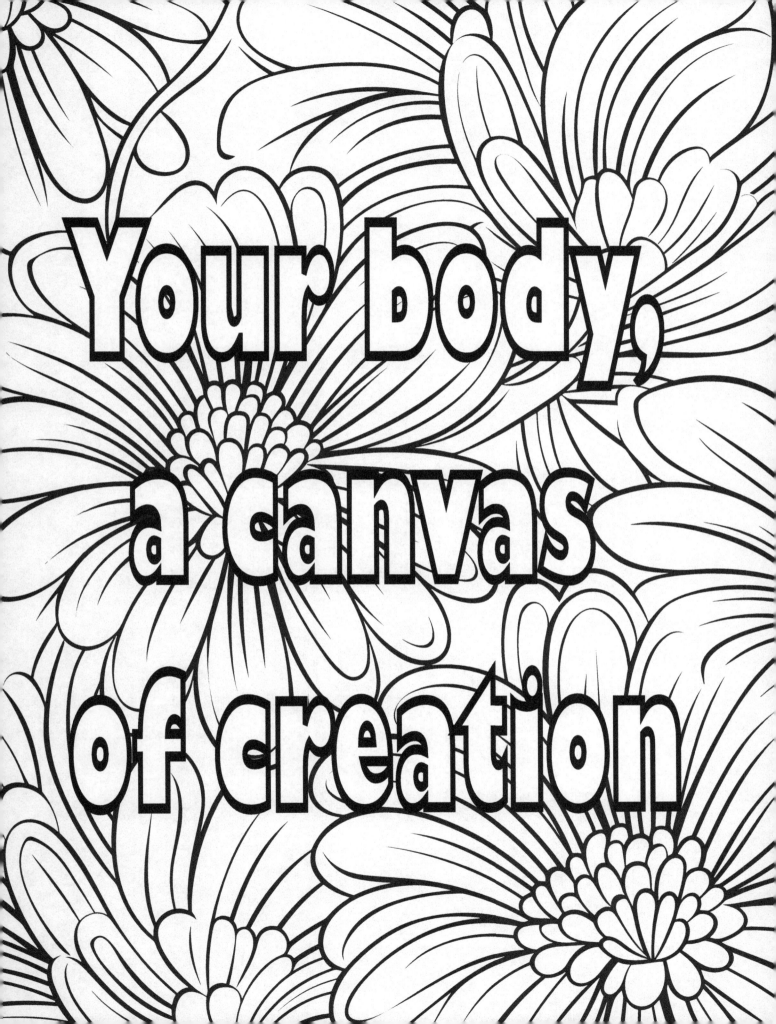

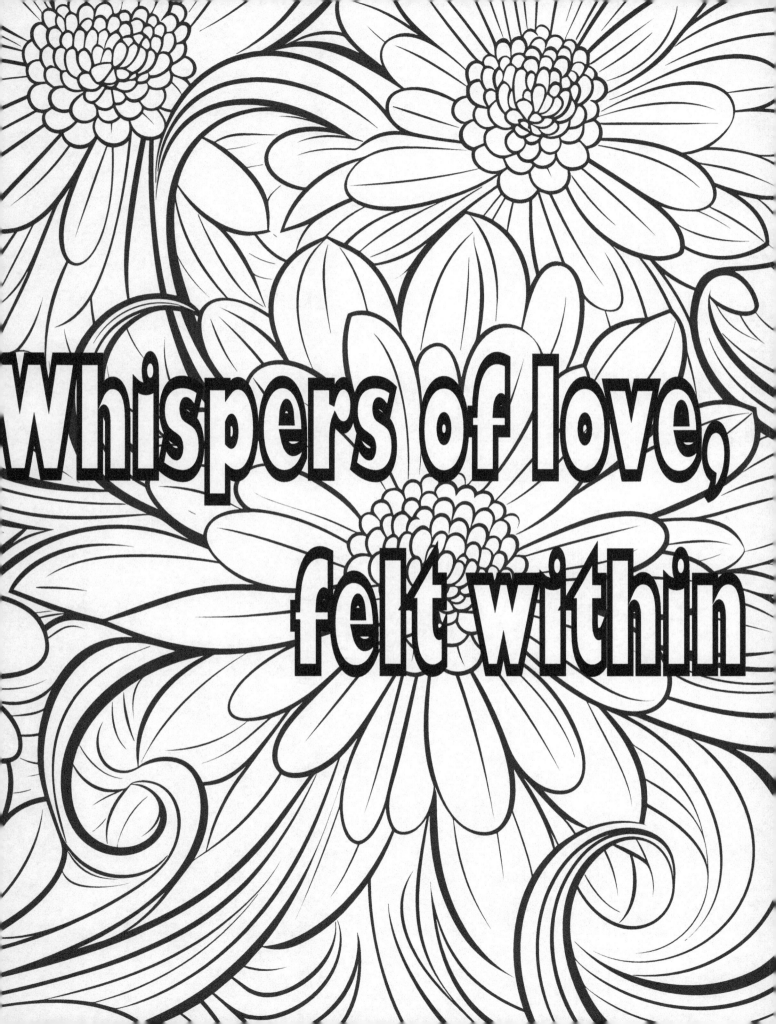

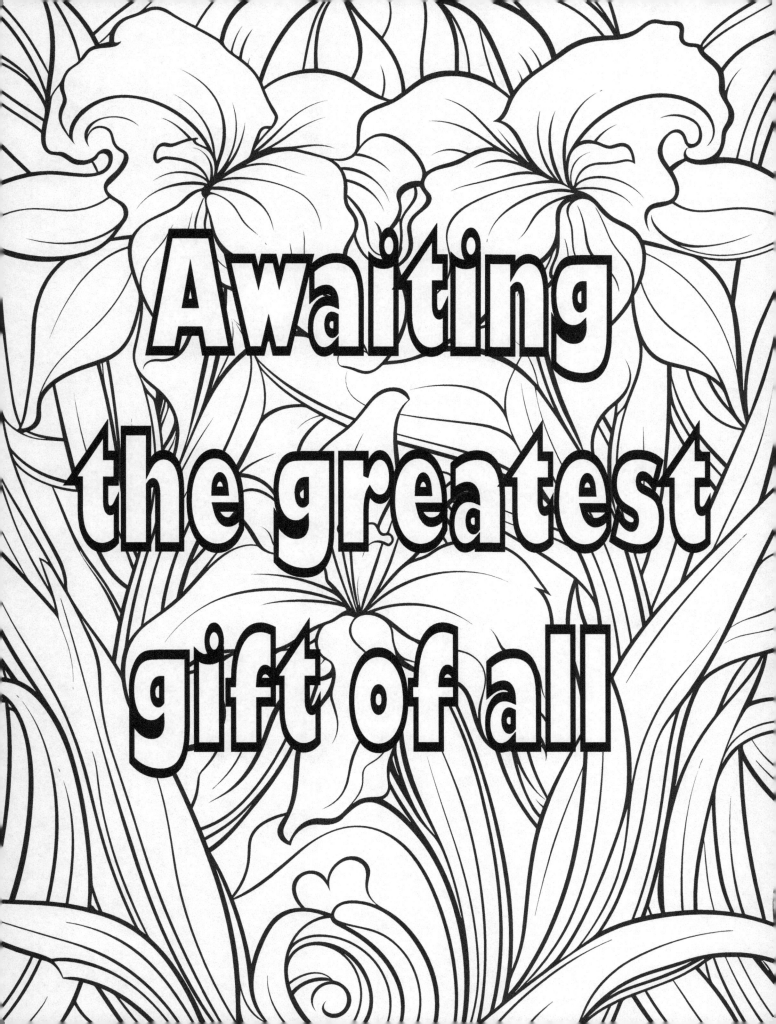

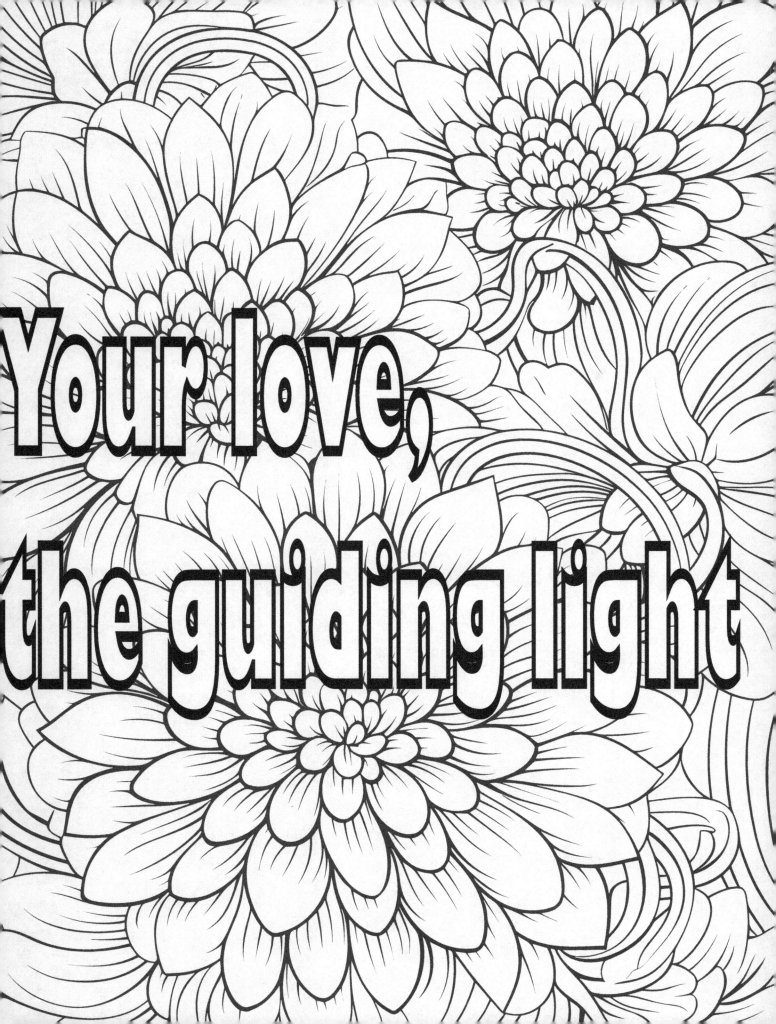

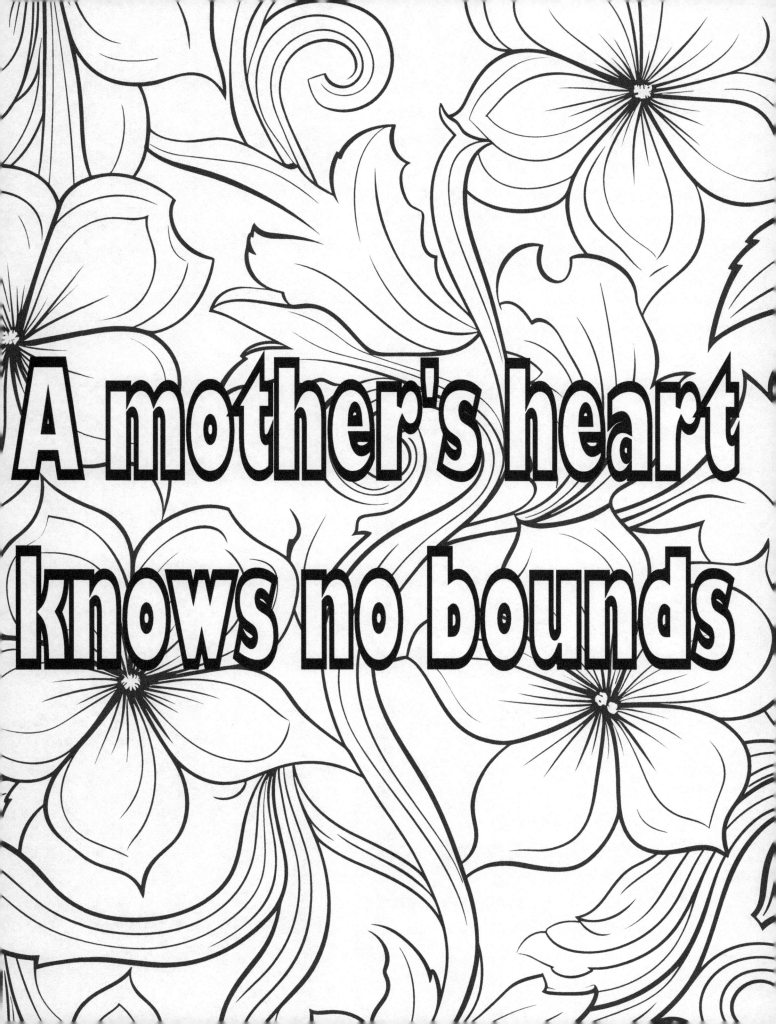

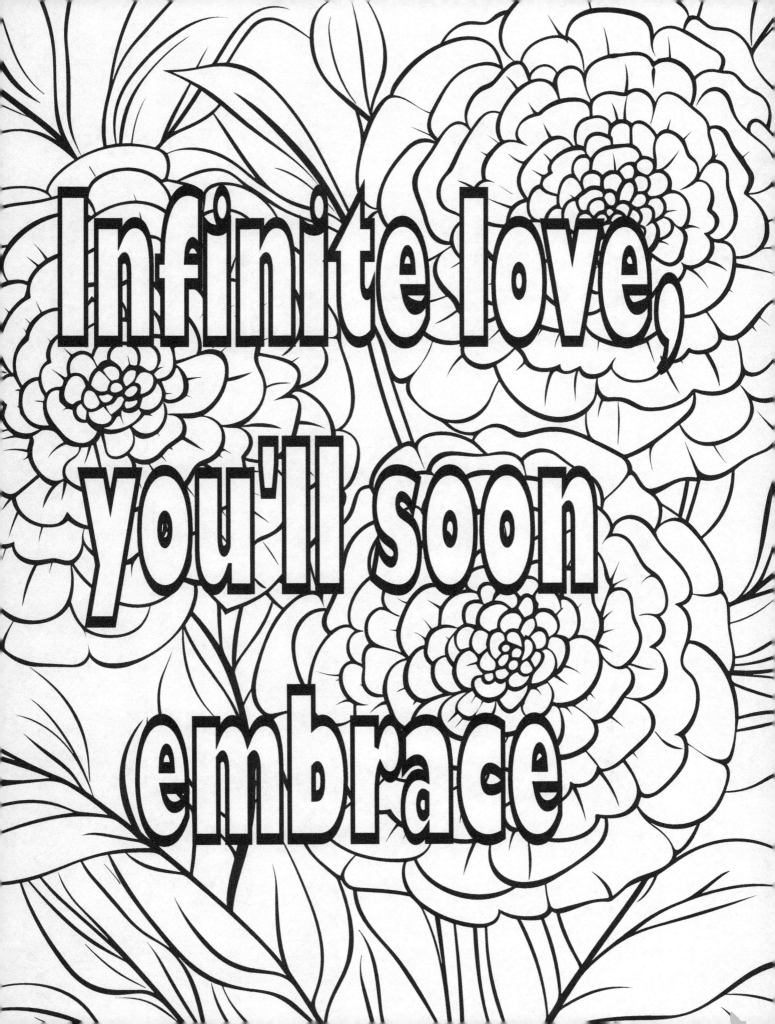

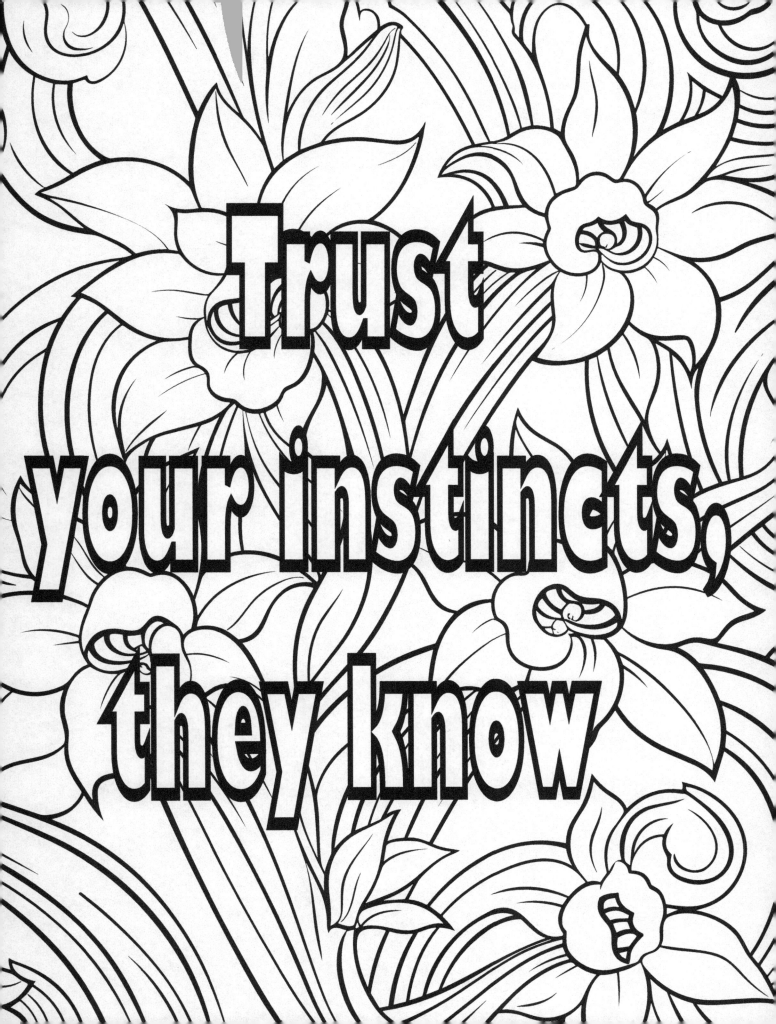

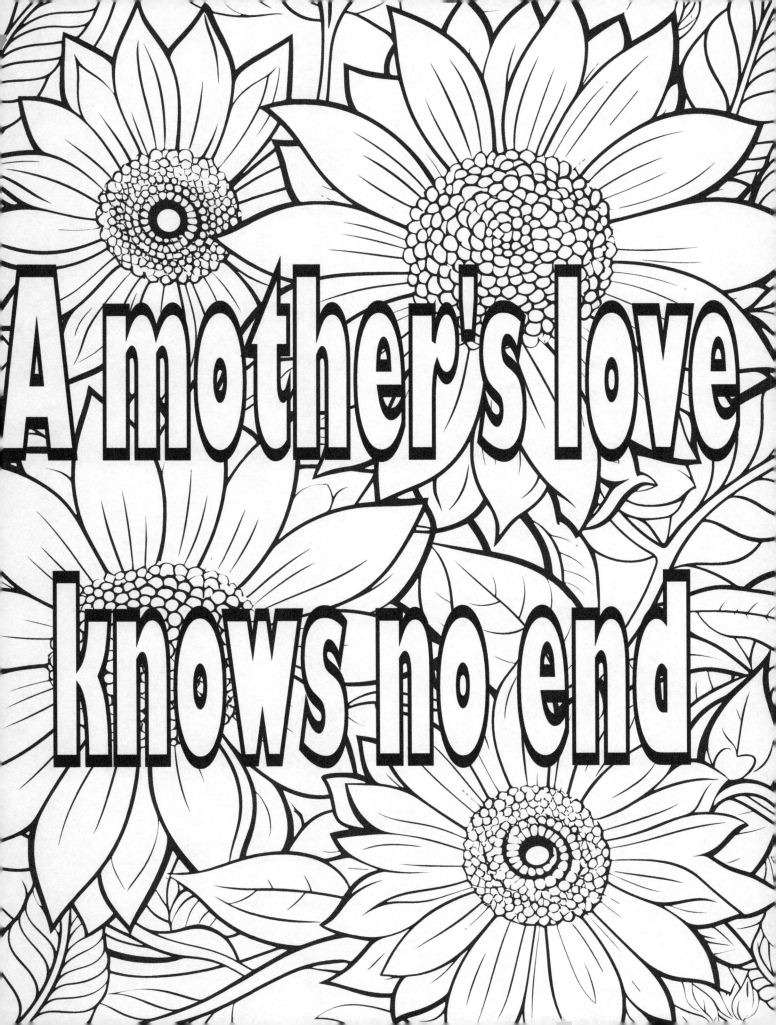

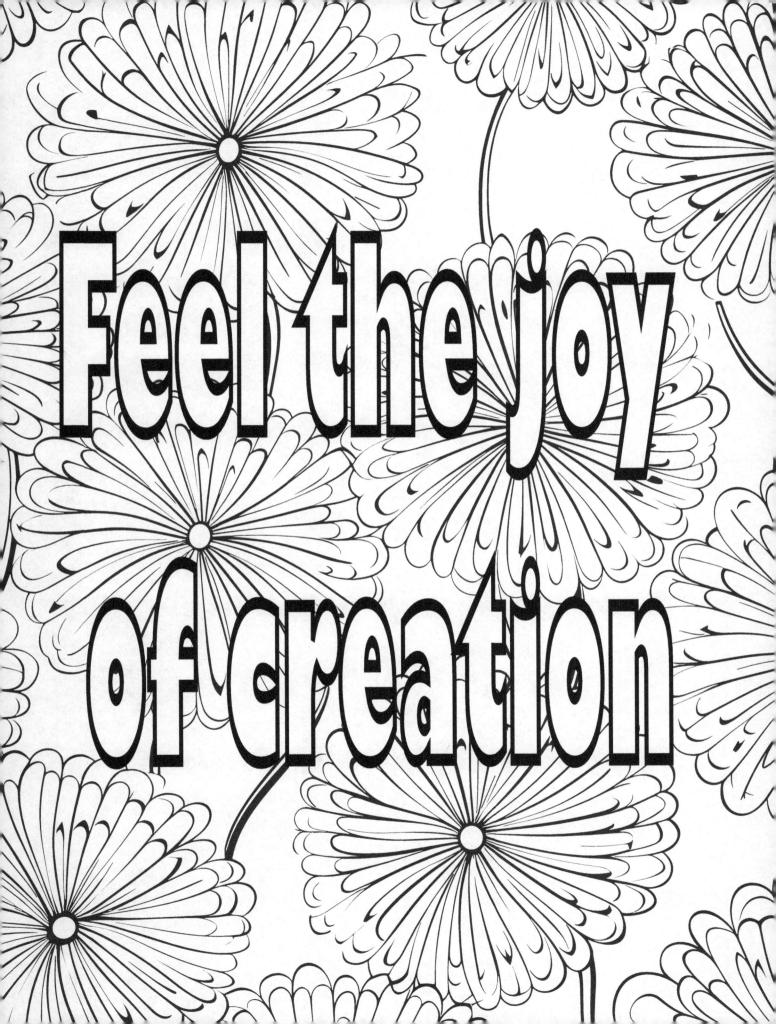

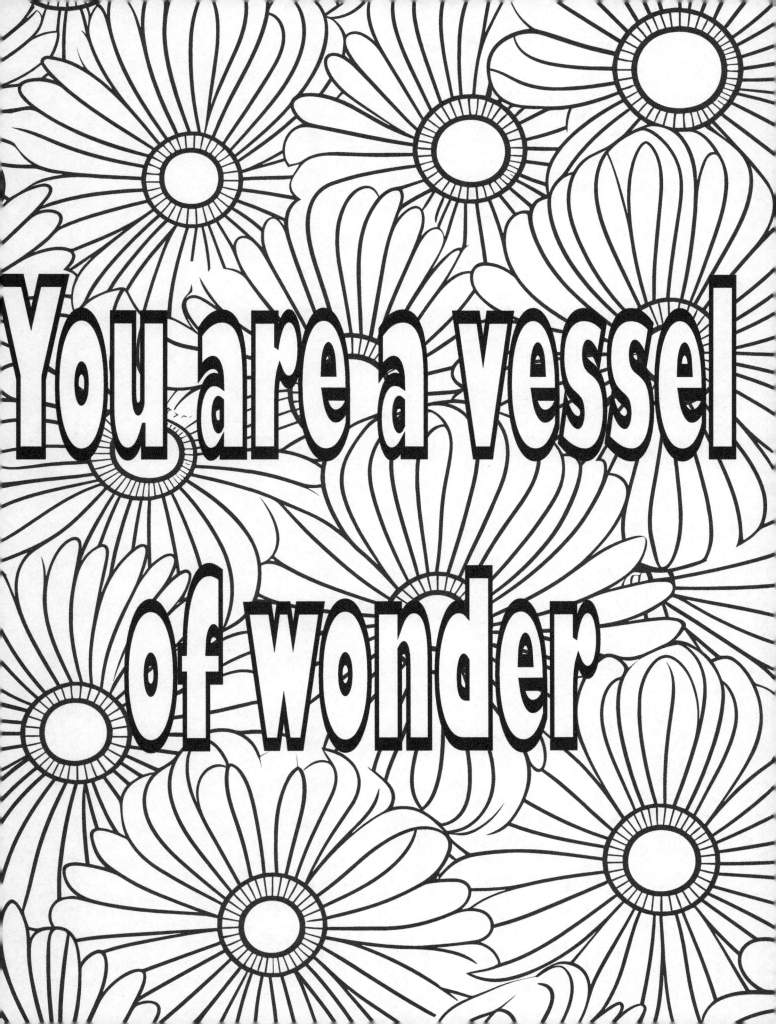

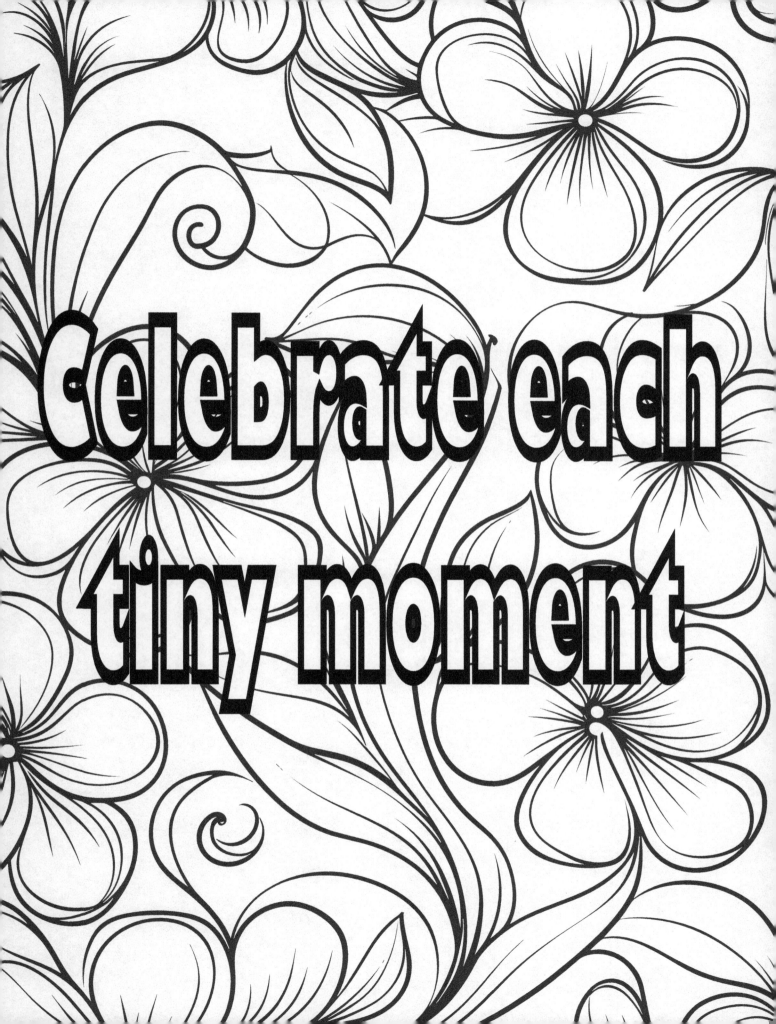

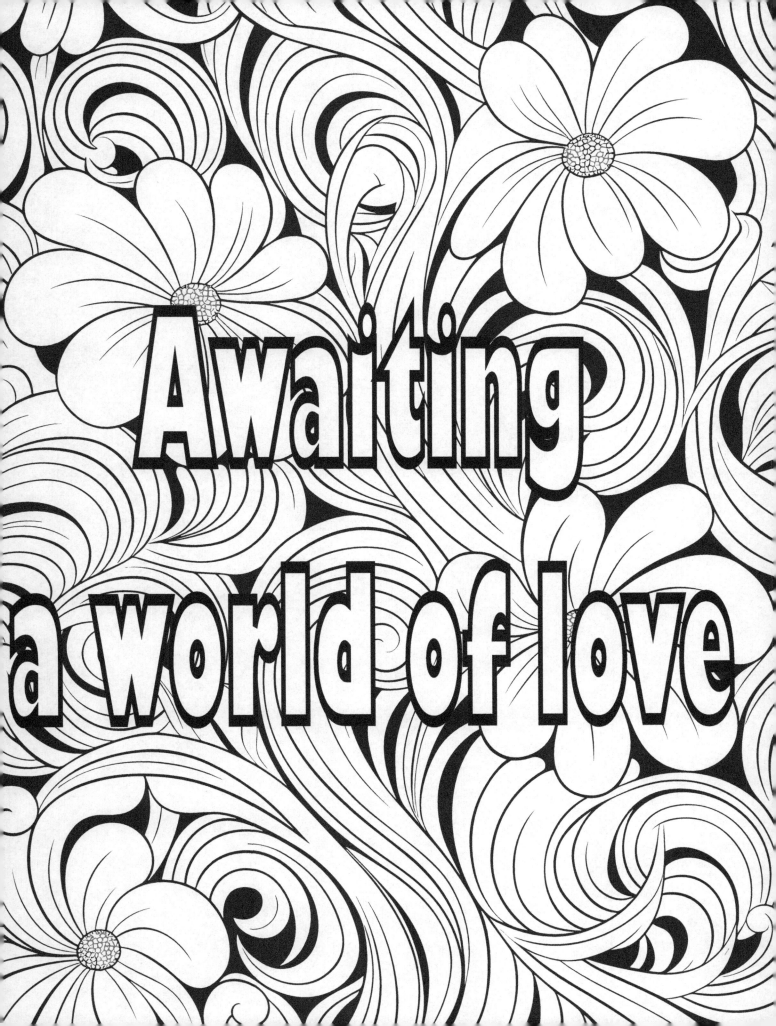

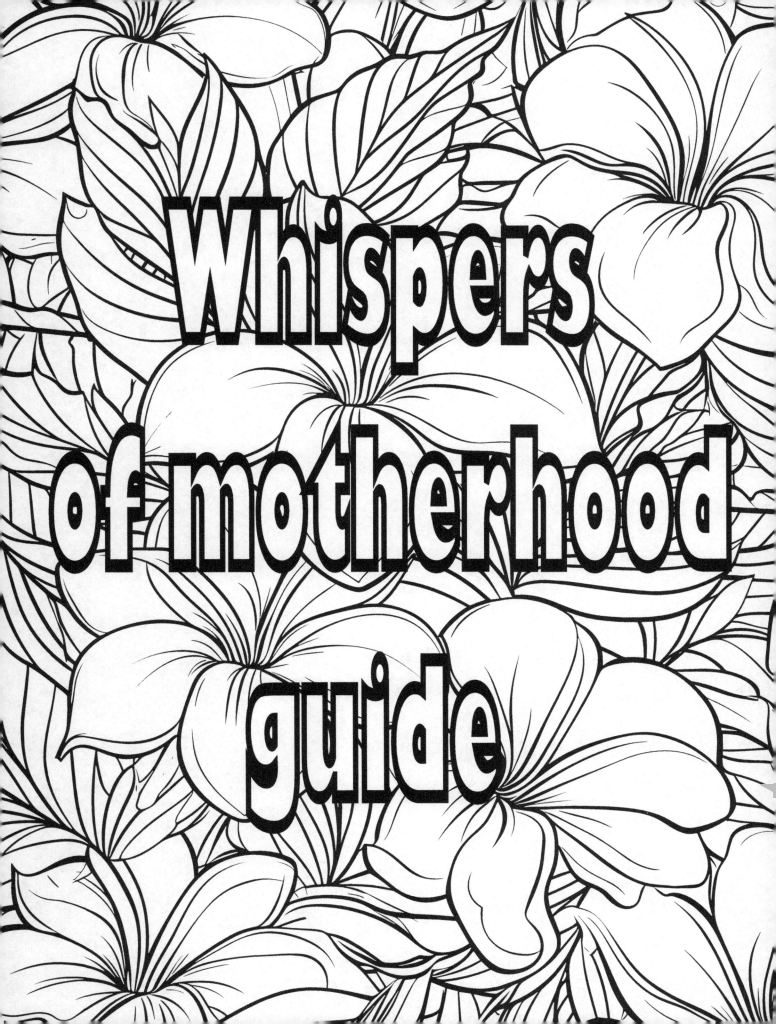

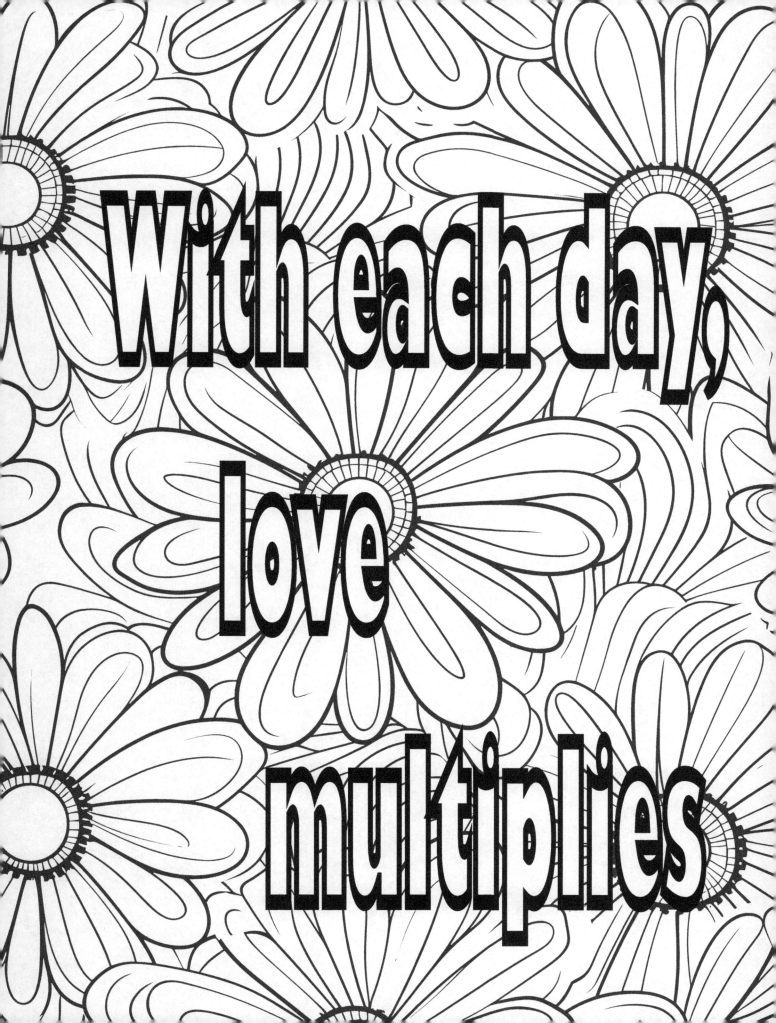

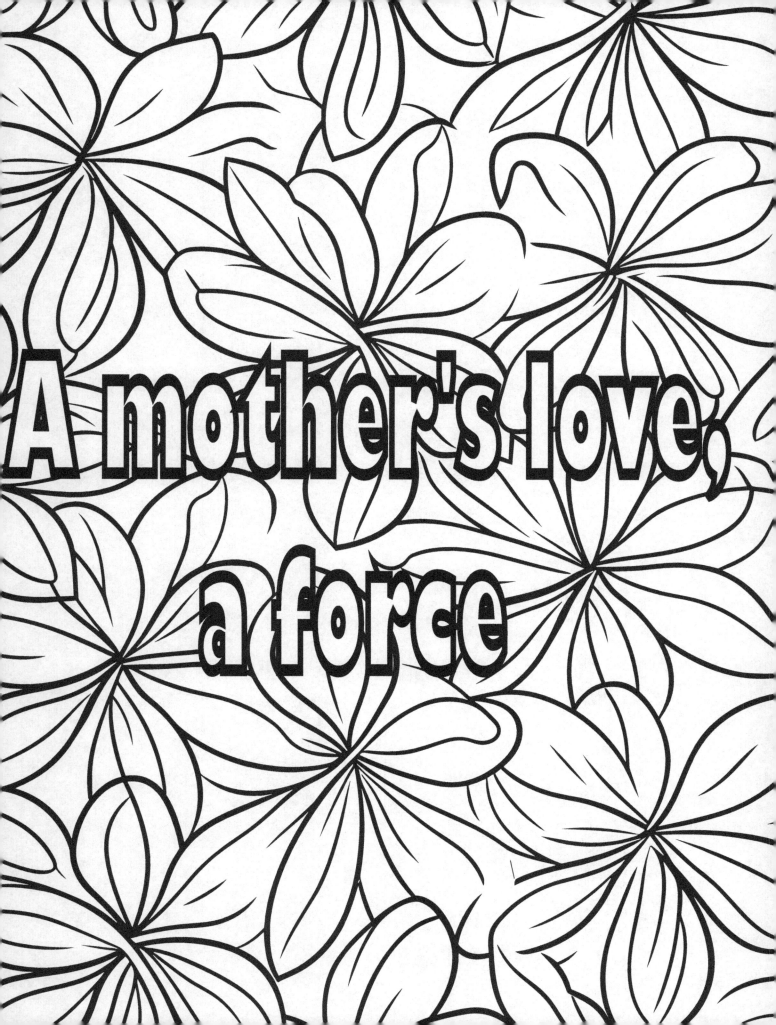

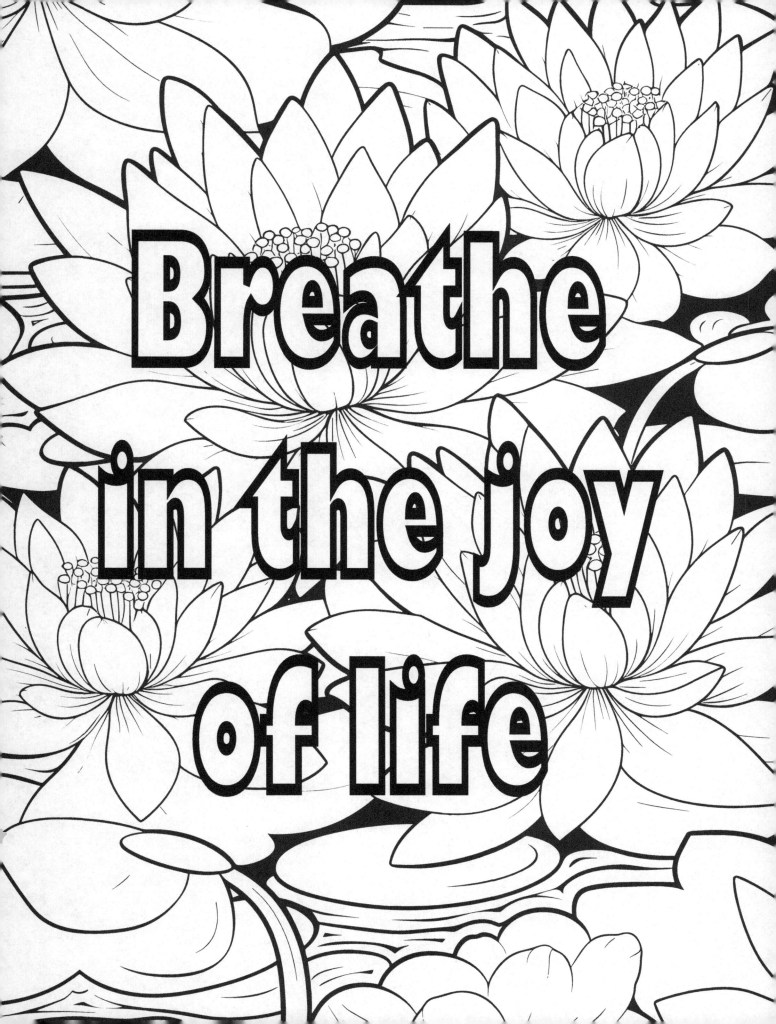

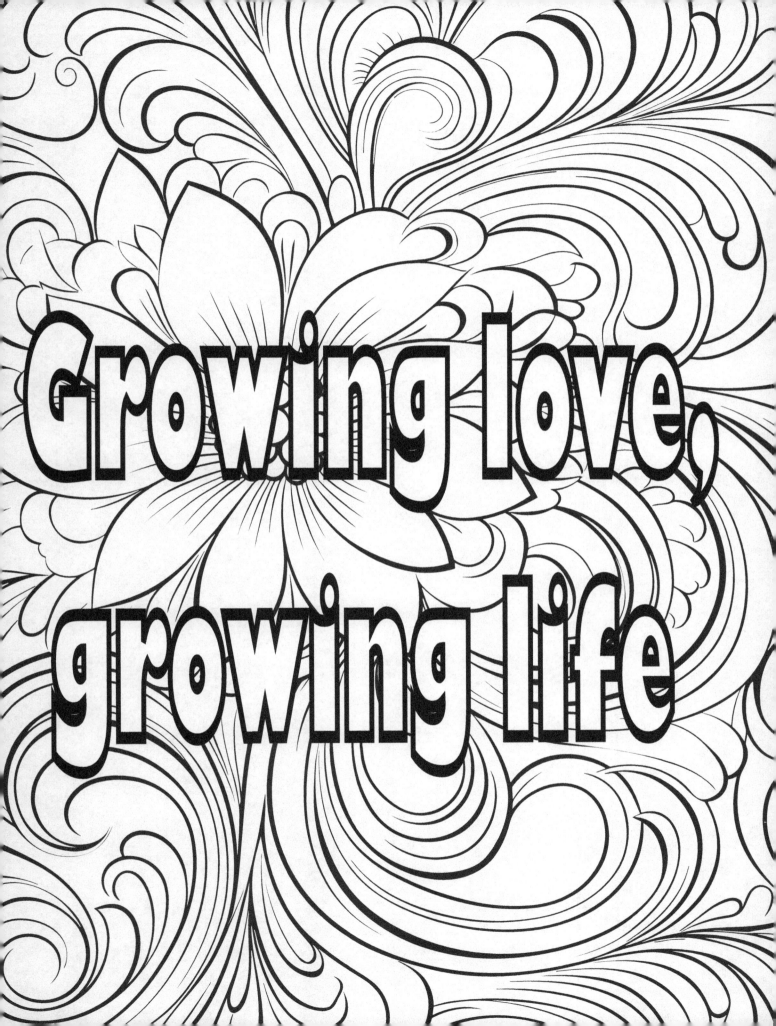

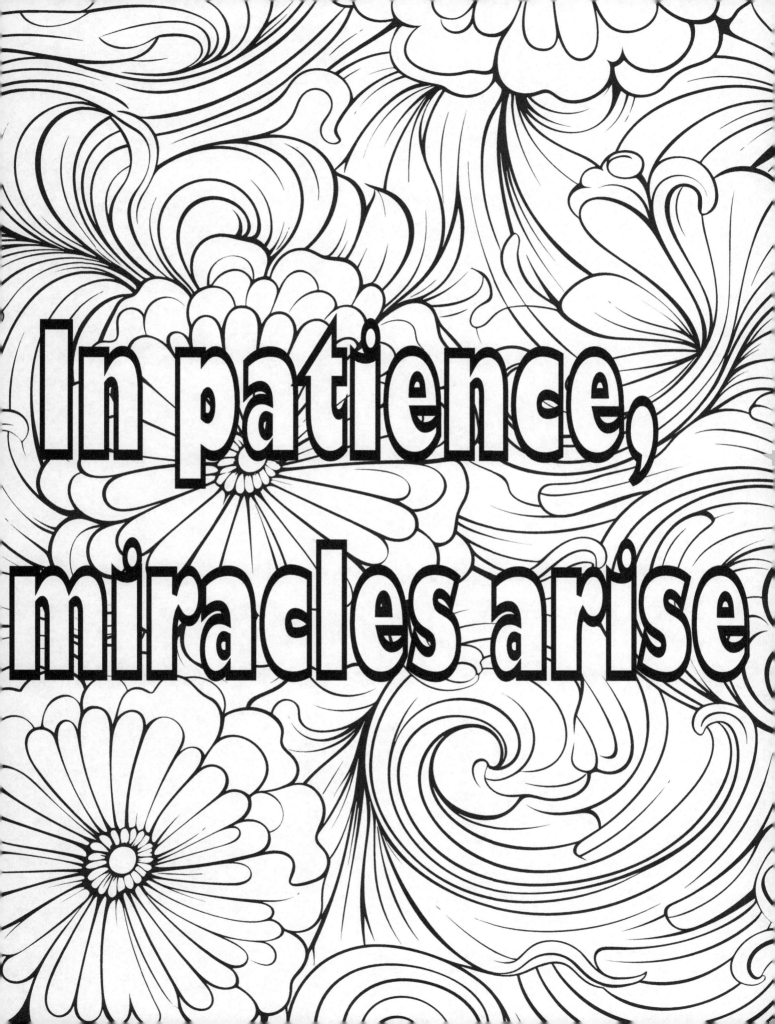

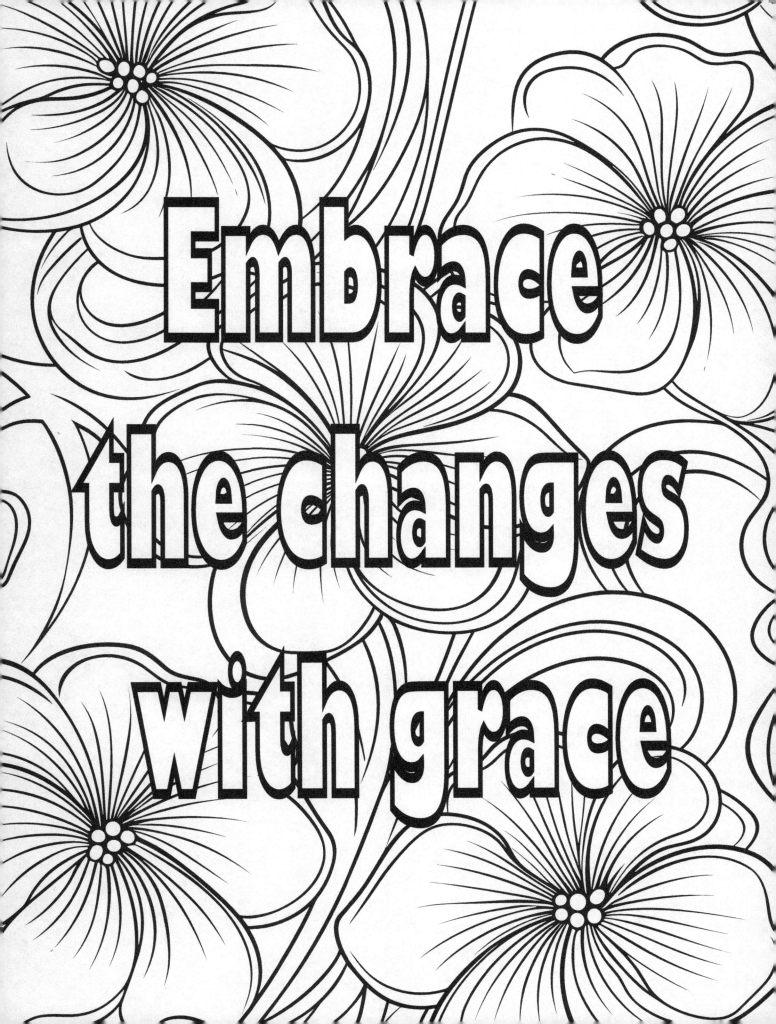

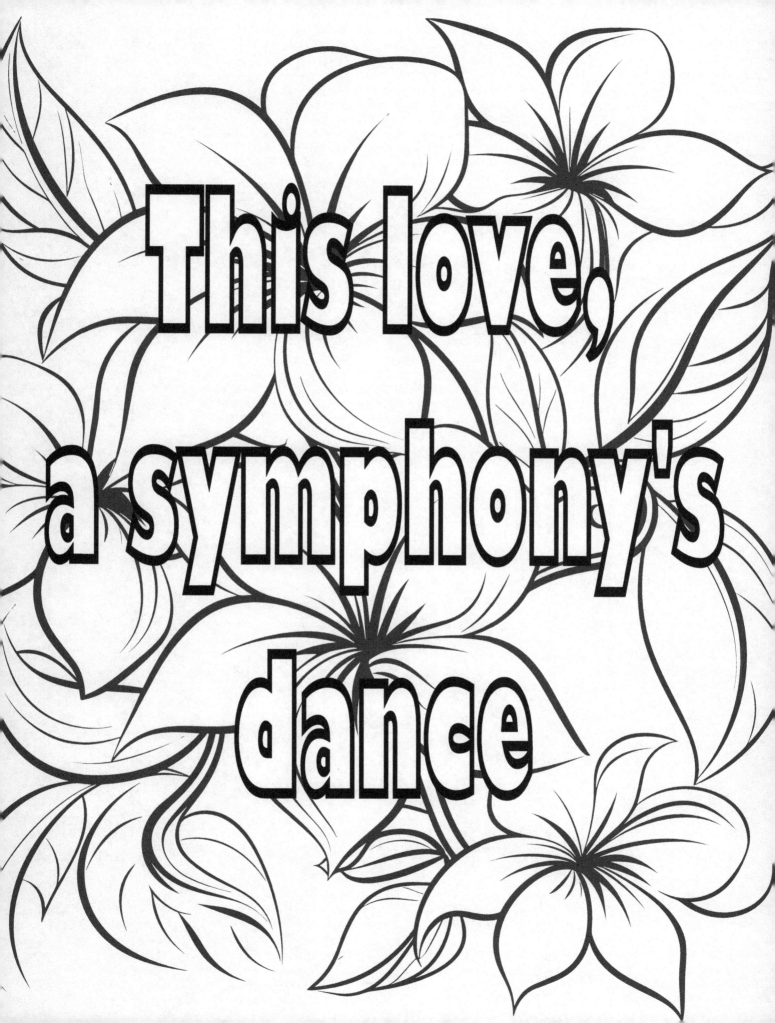

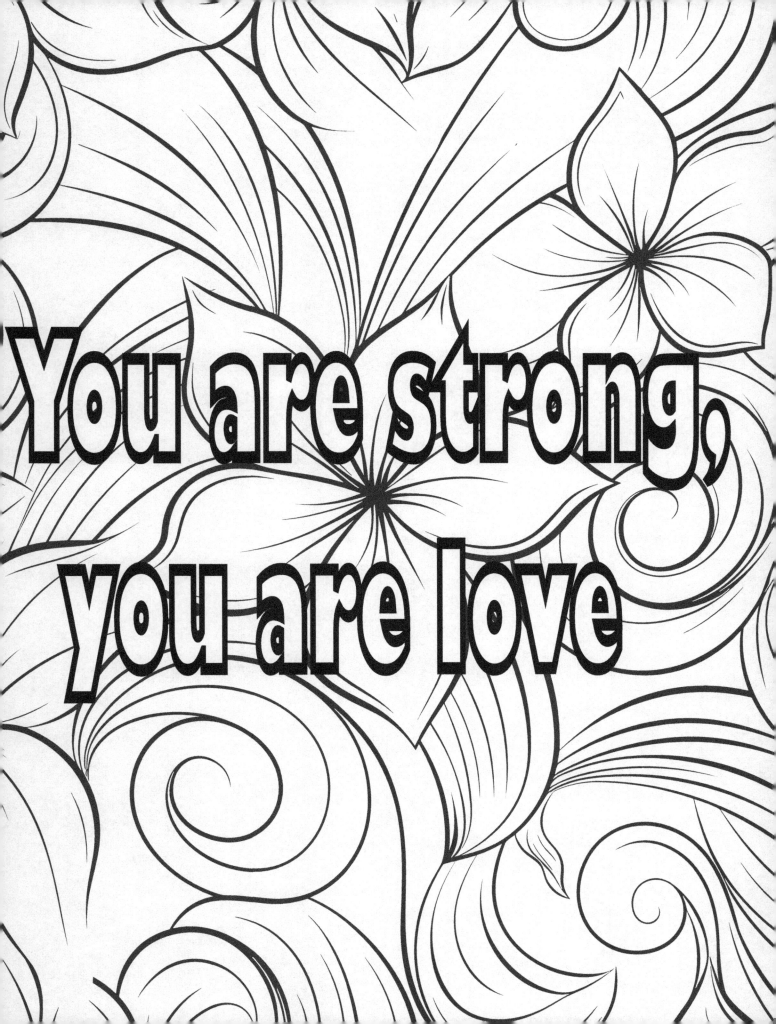

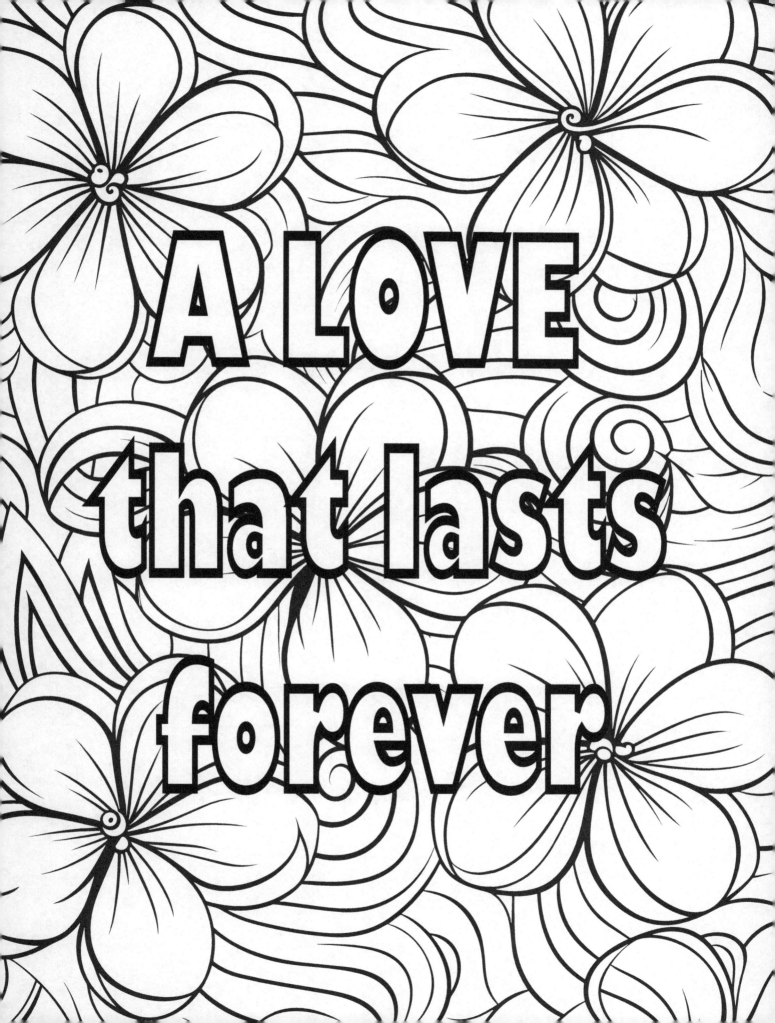

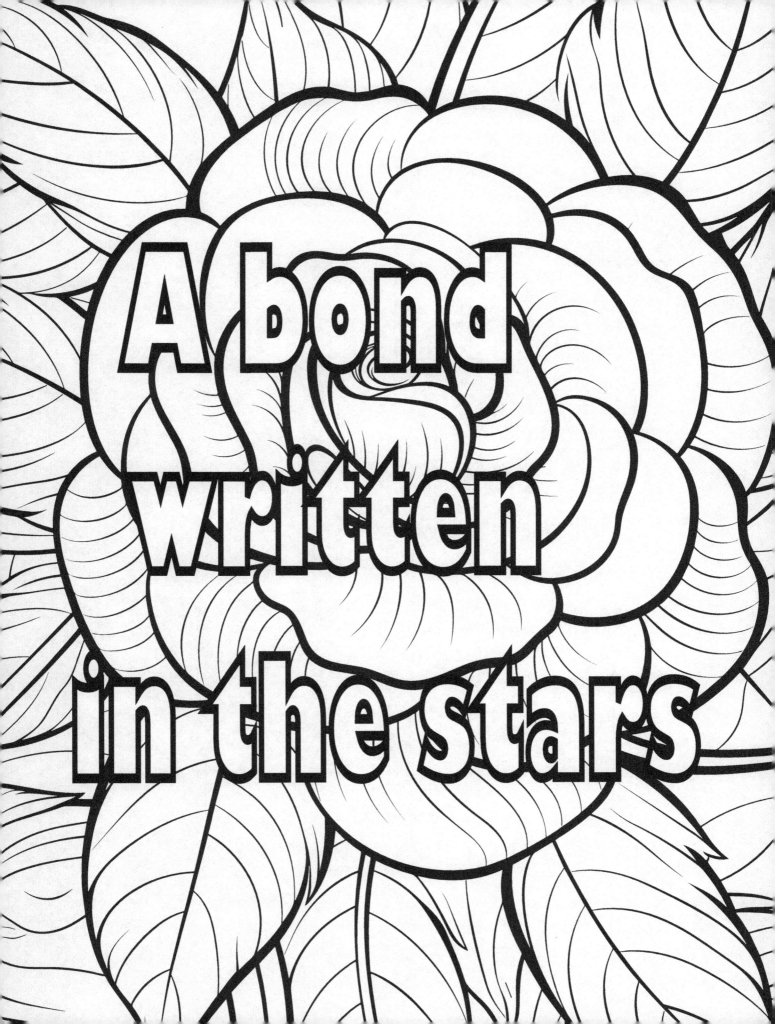

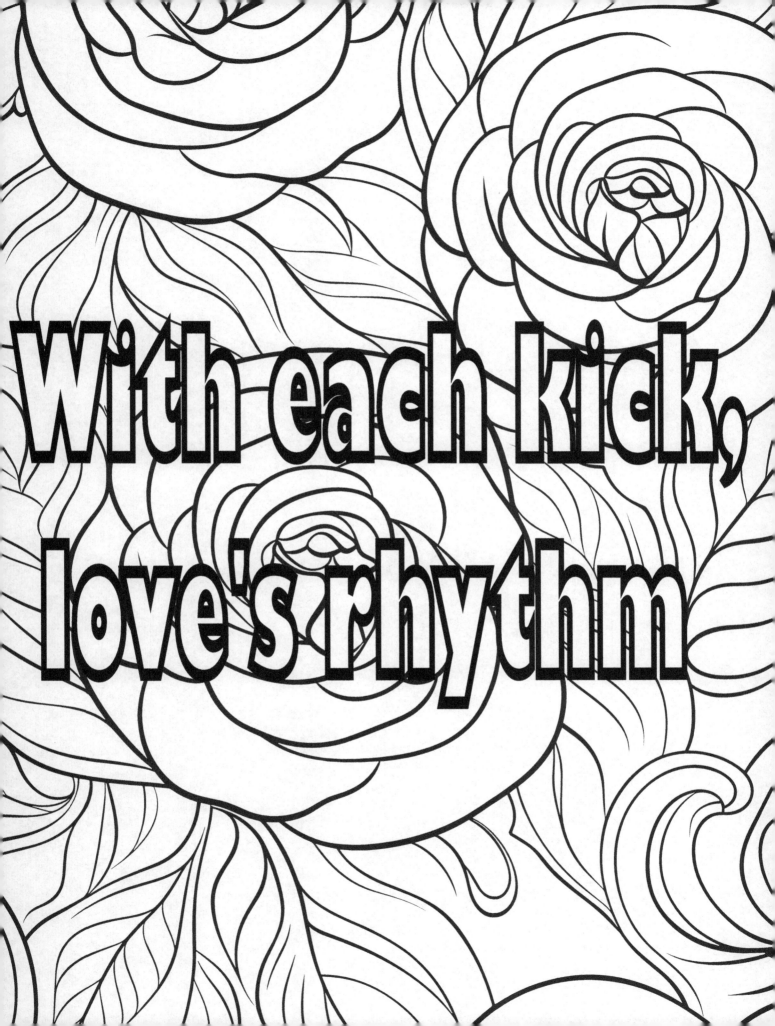

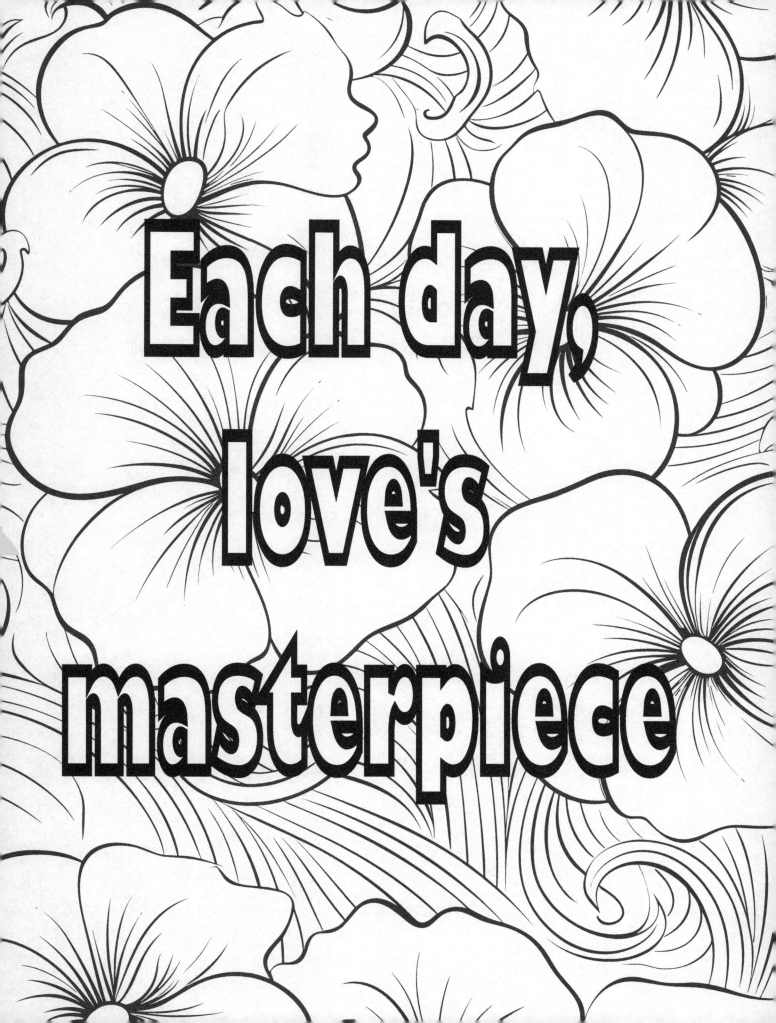

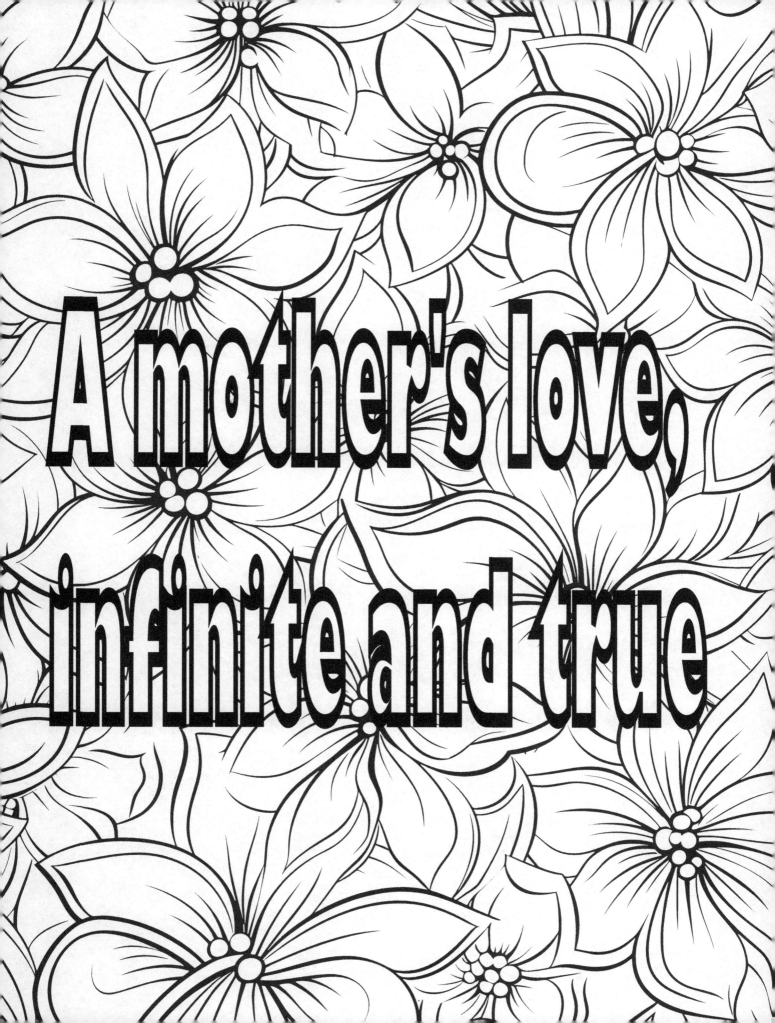

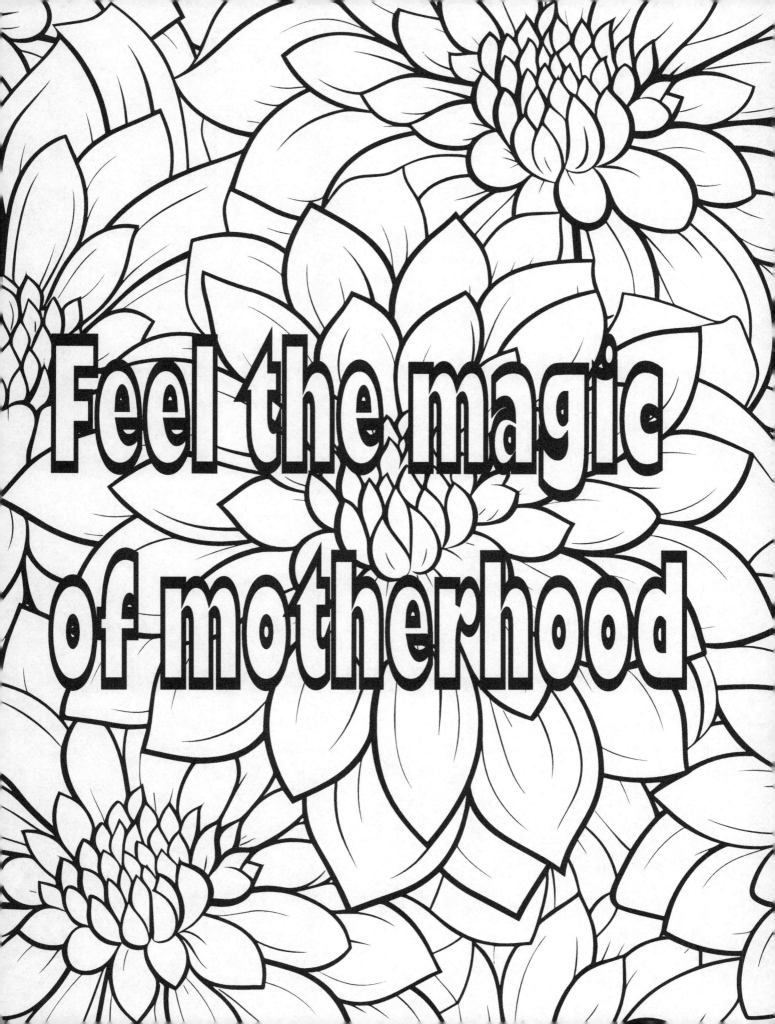

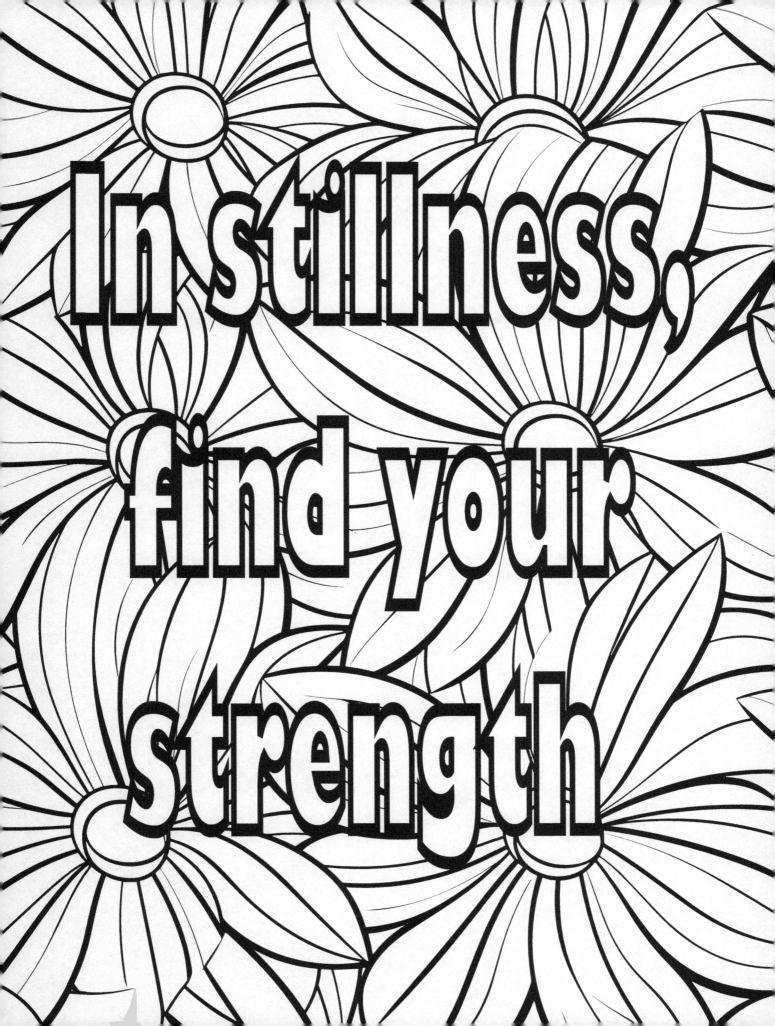

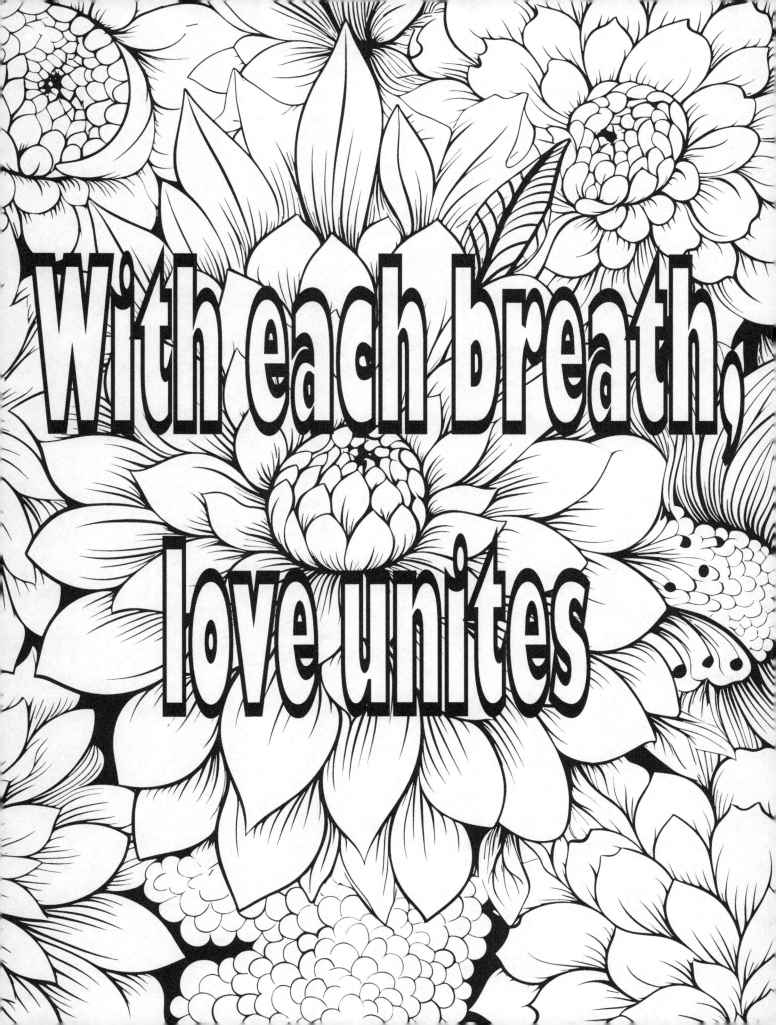

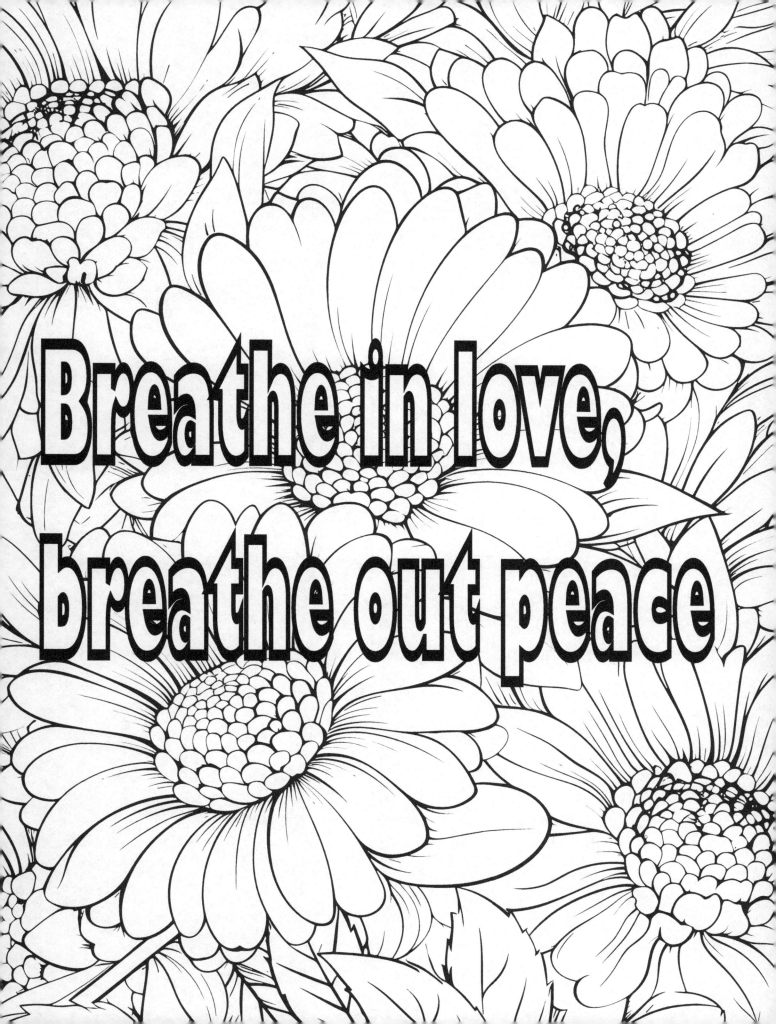

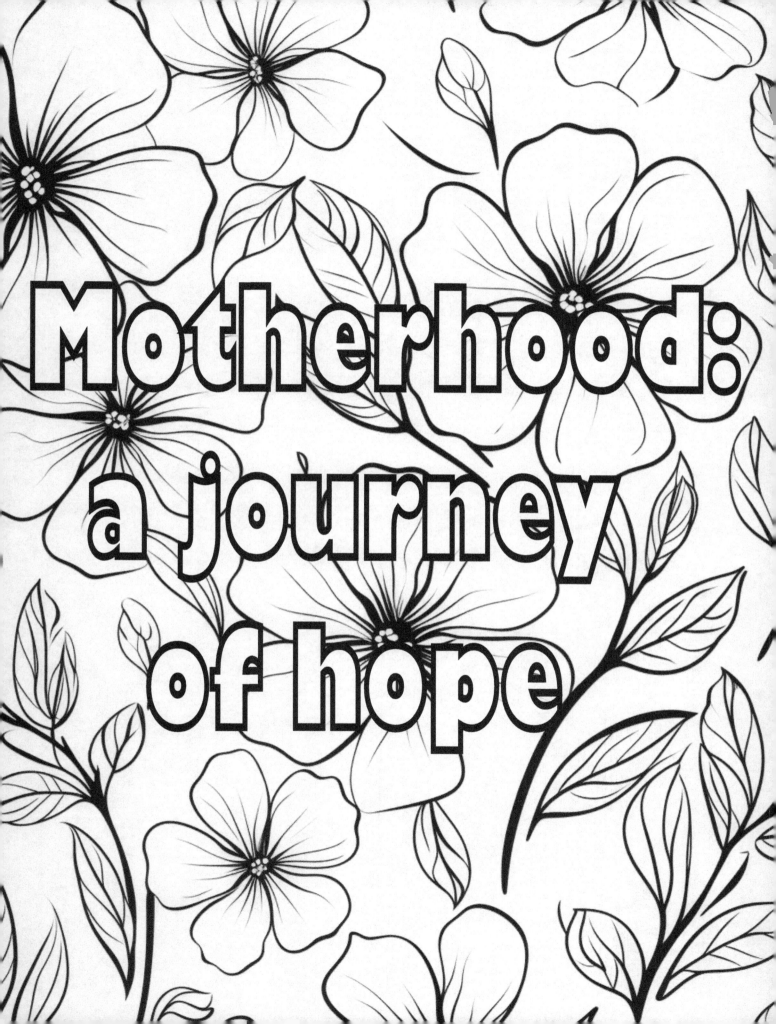

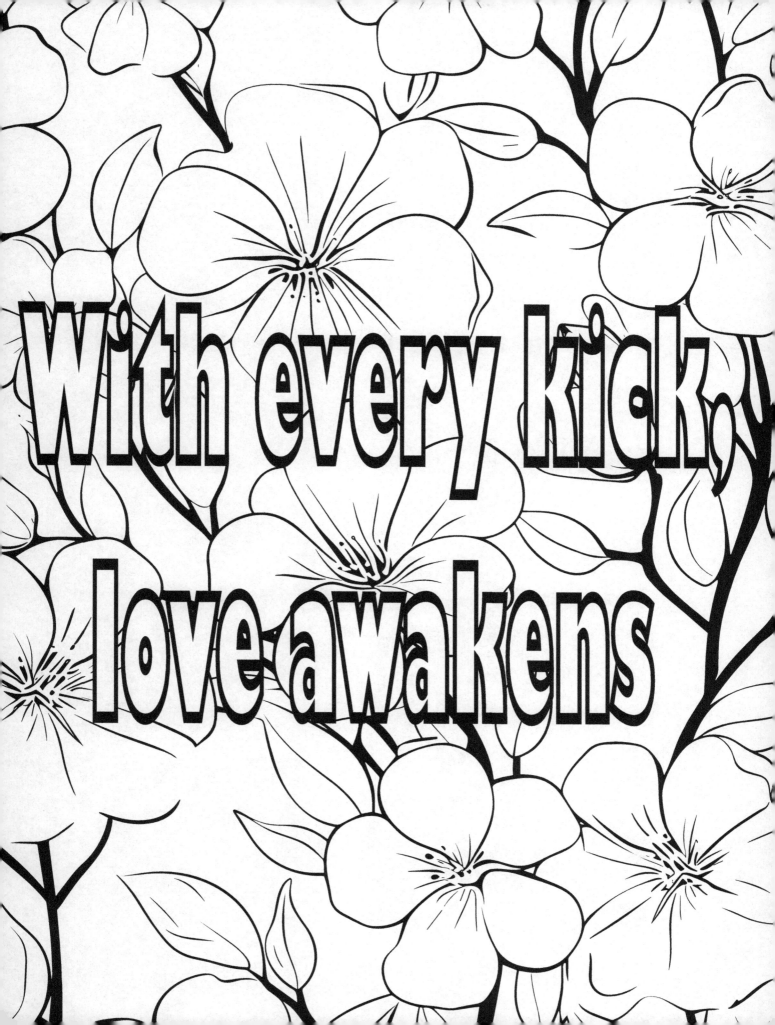

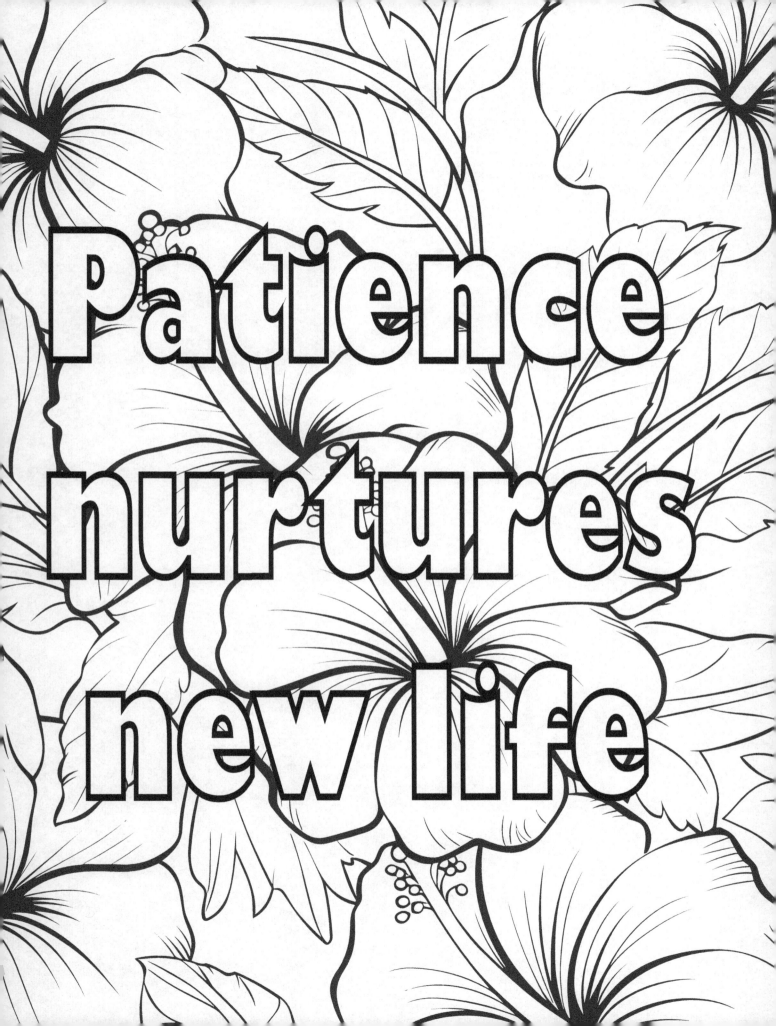

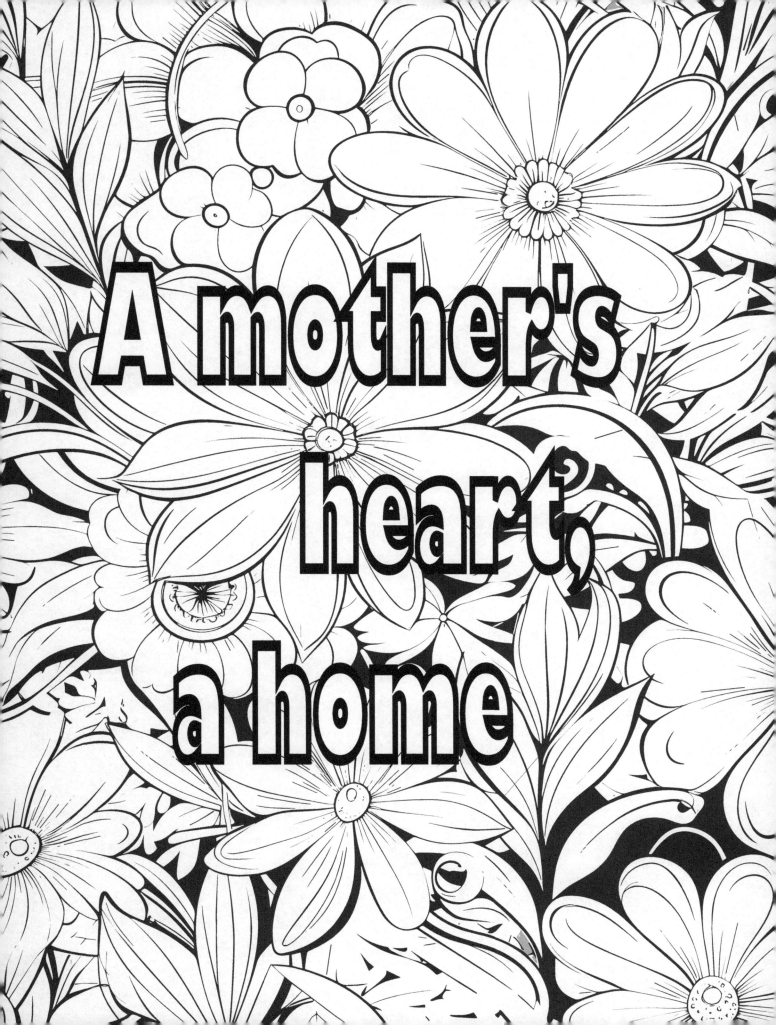

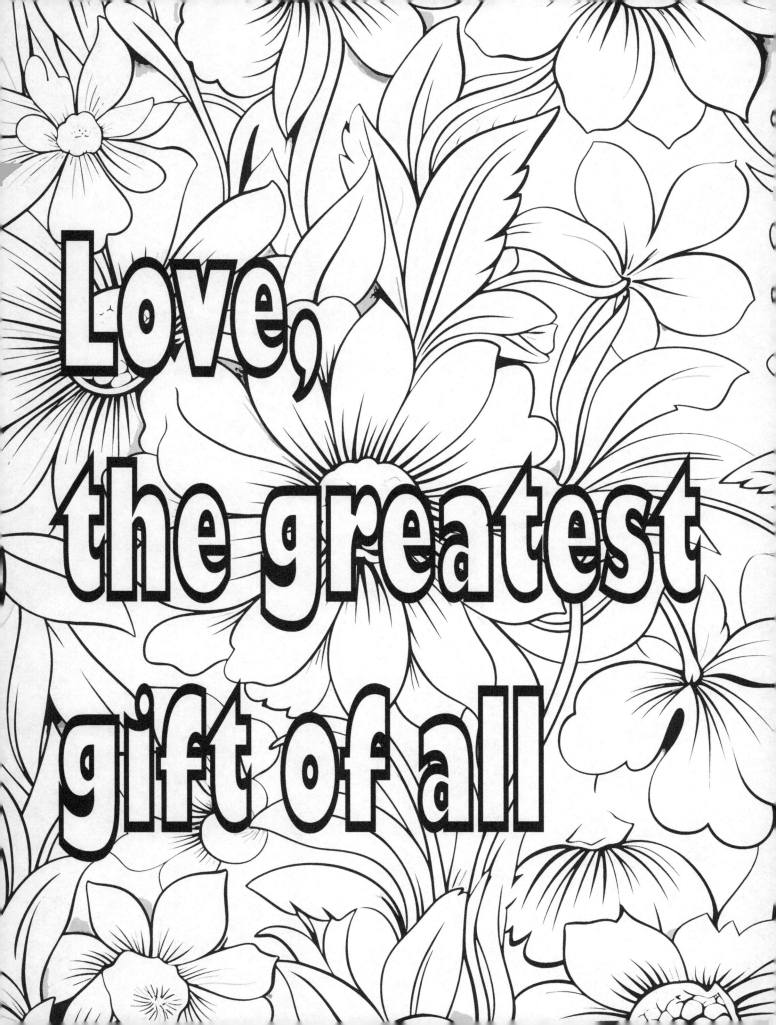

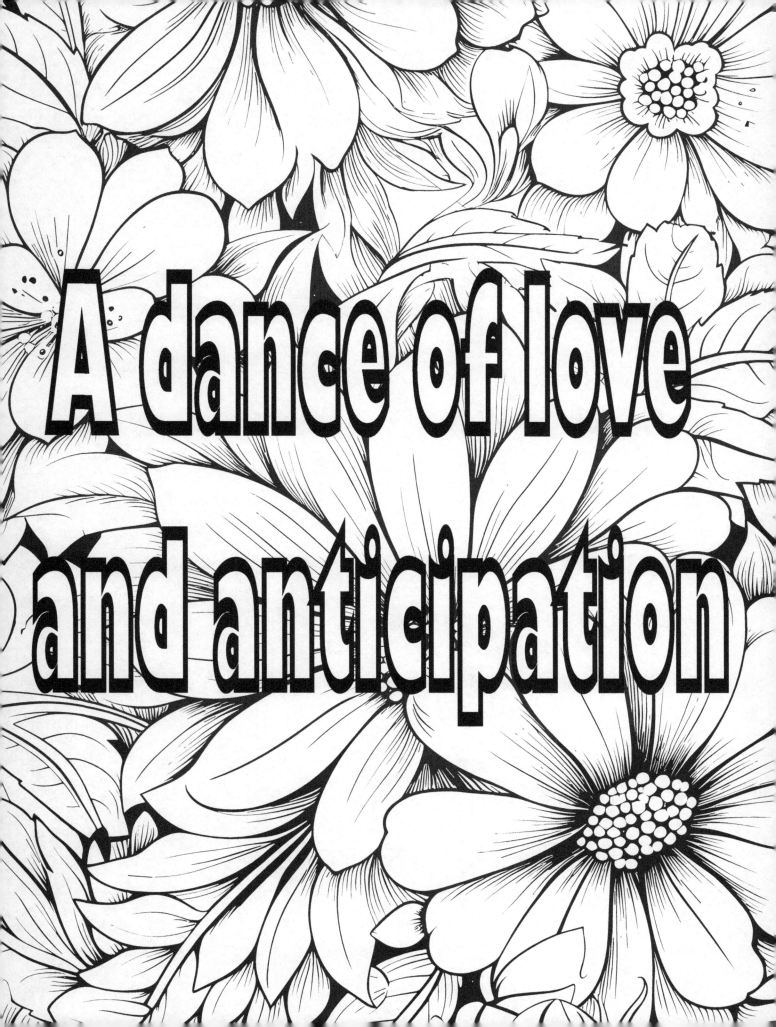

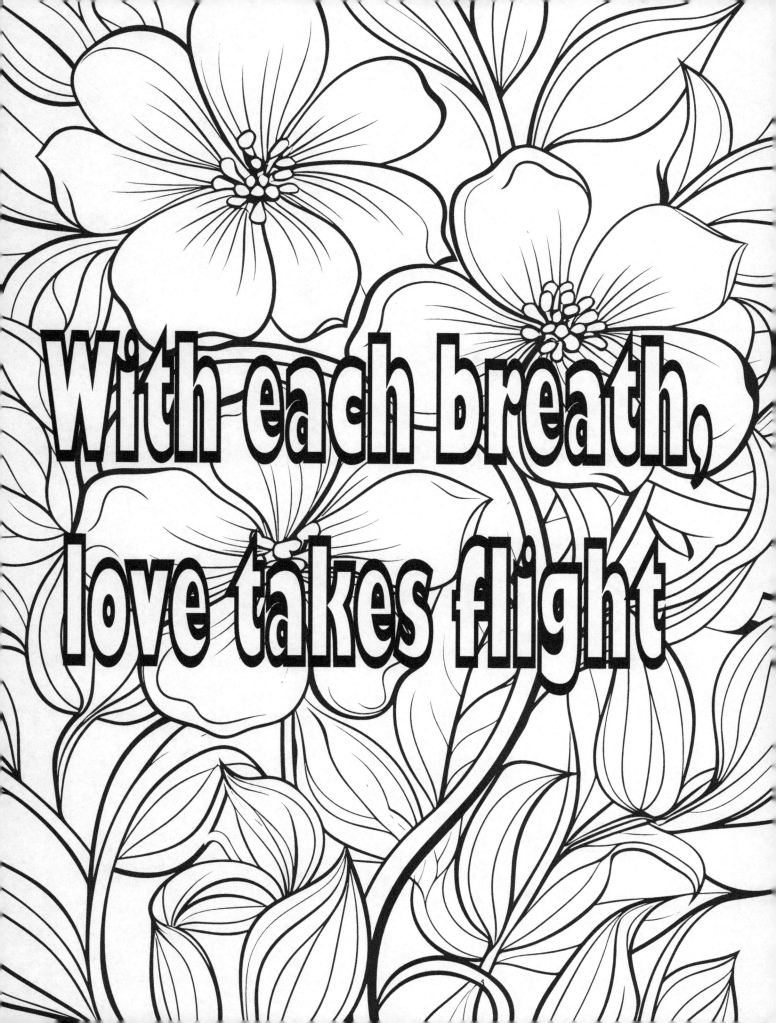

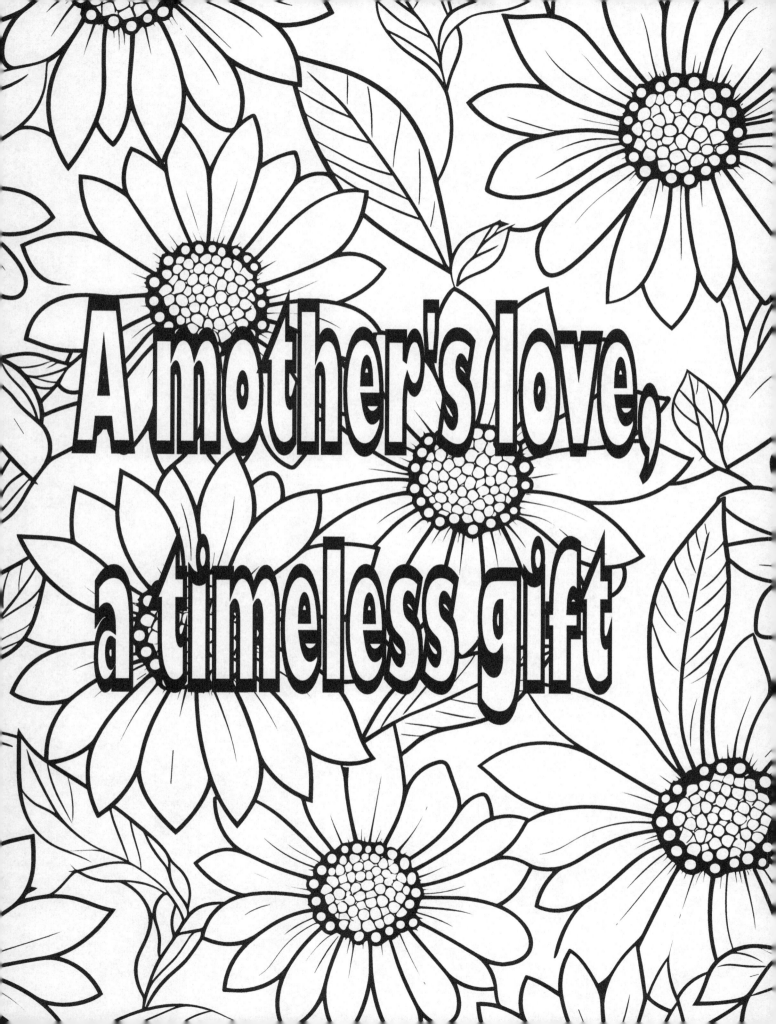

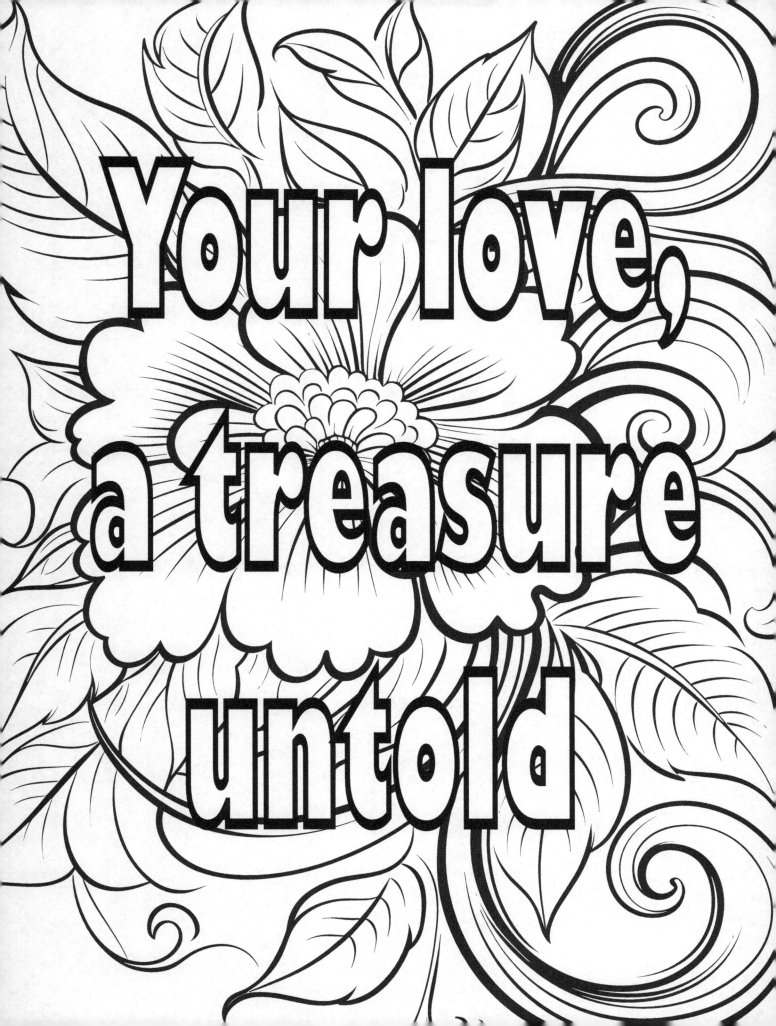

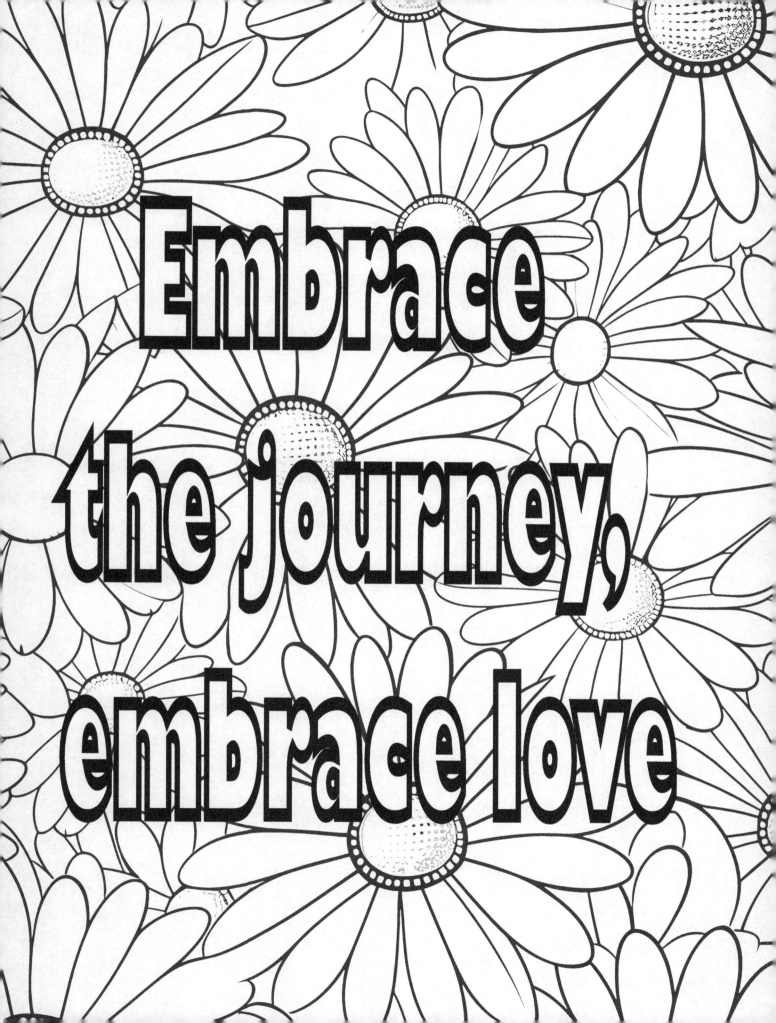

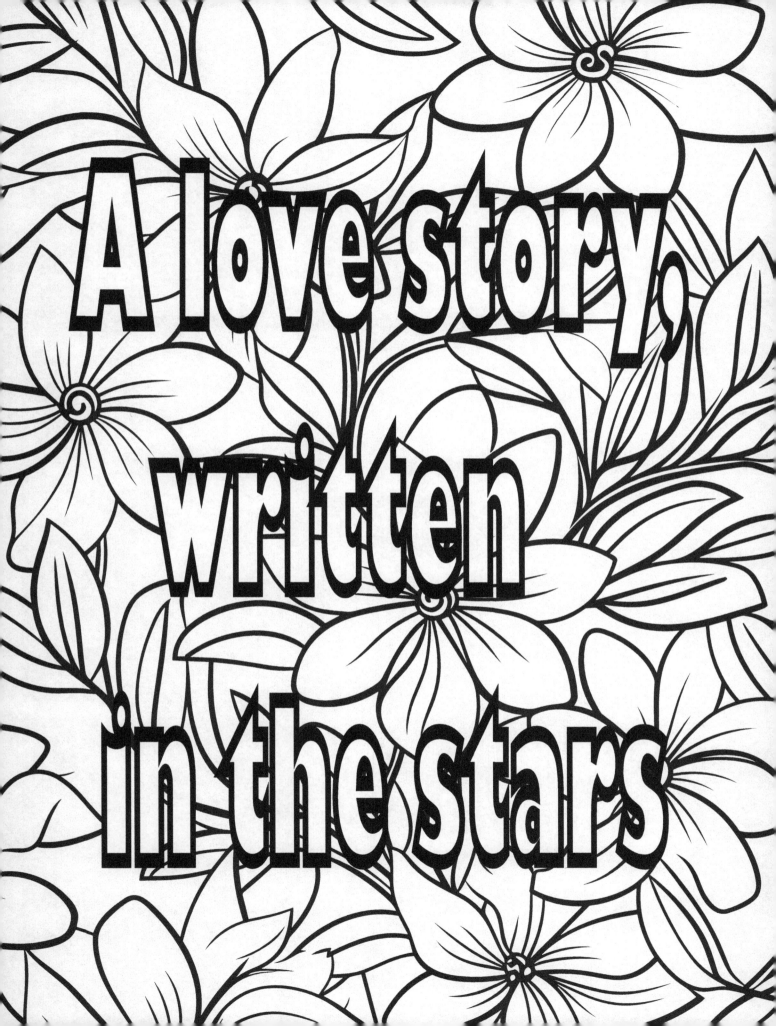

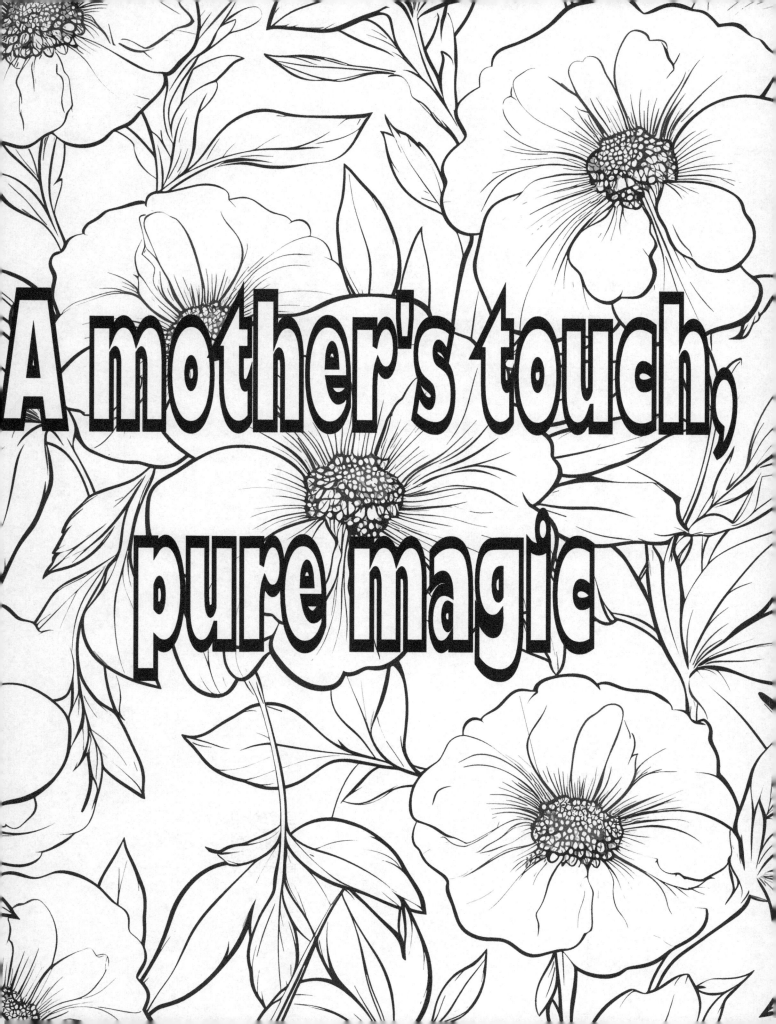

Dear Beautiful Moms-to-Be,

We hope our Quotes Coloring Book has been a source of

relaxation and inspiration during this precious time in your life.

Creating this book was a labor of love, and your thoughts mean the world to us.

If you could take a moment to share your experience with us by leaving a review

on Amazon, it would truly brighten our day and help other expecting moms find

solace in these pages.

Thank you for being a part of our community and for considering this small gesture.

We wish you a smooth and joyful pregnancy filled with colorful moments.

Warm regards,

Stella Booker Publishing

Made in the USA
Las Vegas, NV
26 January 2024

84937776R10057